Prevention

GET SHARPER EVERY DAY

365 Quick & Clever Memory Tricks, Games & More To Boost Your Brain

This book is intended as a reference volume only, not as a medical manual. The information given here is designed to help you make informed decisions about your health. It is not intended as a substitute for any treatment that may have been prescribed by your doctor. If you suspect that you have a medical problem, we urge you to seek competent medical help.

Any mention of specific companies, organizations, or authorities in this book does not imply endorsement by the author or publisher, nor does any mention of specific companies, organizations, or authorities imply that they endorse this book, its author, or the publisher.

Internet addresses and telephone numbers given in this book were accurate at the time it went to press.

© 2021 by Hearst Magazines, Inc.

All rights reserved. No part of this publication may be reproduced or transmitted in any form or by any means, electronic or mechanical, including photocopying, recording, or any other information storage and retrieval system, without the written permission of the publisher.

Prevention is a registered trademark of Hearst Magazines, Inc.

Book design by Lauren Vitello | Illustrations by TheNounProject

Library of Congress Cataloging-in-Publication Data is on file with the publisher.

ISBN 978-1-950099-96-2

Printed in China

2 4 6 8 10 9 7 5 3 1 paperback

HEARST

Prevention

GET SHARPER EVERY DAY

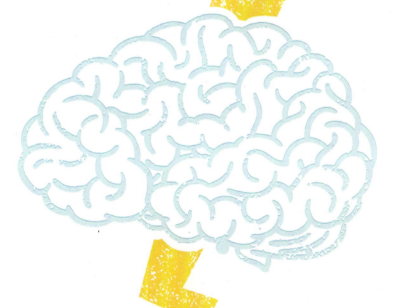

365 Quick & Clever Memory Tricks, Games & More To Boost Your Brain

HOW THIS BOOK WORKS

Let's face it, who doesn't want to be a little faster mentally, concentrate better, sleep better, know more, live longer, and remember your mom's best friend's dog's birthday? Whether you're 28 or 82, this book contains ways to improve your brainpower—often while also improving your physical well-being, verbal skills, peace of mind, and sense of wonder.

In these pages you'll find daily tips to enrich your brain through physical, mental, and nutrition strategies, along with memory hacks and games. One thing you won't be? Bored. We've selected the best ideas from the pages of our magazine and previous books, with plenty of insightful advice from top-tier experts. Here are the categories you'll find in this book, and why we're including them:

 GAME SMART

Mounting scientific evidence suggests that people who constantly challenge their minds to solve problems and absorb new information have the sharpest, clearest, and hardest-working minds. Scientists have long held the belief that problem-solving activities like crossword puzzles can improve brain function and protect the mind from cognitive decline later in life. As well, a variety of challenges helps keep your mind on its synapses.

So keep your brain busy. Do crossword and Sudoku puzzles. Read interesting books. Play Scrabble. Virtually any activity that keeps your mind active may help reduce your risk of age-related memory decline. In this book we've provided lots of games (and the answers on page 329) to keep you busy for an entire year.

BRAIN SMART

Your brain is like any other body part. A few gym workouts might have your biceps or quads feeling firmer and tighter, but you have to make a habit of exercise to keep them that way. We'll provide useful tips to help stretch your attention span. When you stick to regular gym workouts, you reap a major payoff: preserving those toned muscles you worked so hard to build up. You can do the same thing for your brain.

Fascinating research reveals that regular exercise for your mind helps keep your basic brain skills in shape. This means you think faster, learn more easily, and forget less. In fact, several studies have shown that people who regularly take part in mind-challenging activities—what we like to think of as giving your brain a good stretch—appear to gain impressive protection against dementia.

We'll provide brain-smart tips for learning new information, improving your attention and concentration, enhancing your problem-solving prowess (which is related to creativity), and honing your focus and mental energy.

 ## NUTRITION SMART

We'll suggest easy ways to get your brain food (nutrients, that is) through your meals, many of which are found in the MIND diet. The MIND diet—which stands for "Mediterranean-DASH Intervention for Neurodegenerative Delay"—could not be more aptly named. In one study, researchers found that this eating plan reduced the risk of Alzheimer's disease by 53% among strict adherents, and by 35% among those who followed it "pretty well." We'll introduce you to the MIND diet right away, on Day 3.

We'll also suggest ways to cut down on sugar. Dementia risk increases in people with type 2 diabetes, but even people without diabetes who simply have elevated blood sugar levels may be at increased risk for cognitive decline. That's possibly because of sugar's inflammatory effects on the brain.

 MEMORY SMART

In this book, we'll provide simple, practical mind-sharpening techniques that you can learn in a few minutes. (Some date back to the ancient Greeks!) Once you get the hang of them, the information you need to remember—like the name of that guy you just met at a cocktail party—will stick better. We'll show you some memory tricks and hacks to learn and practice so you can more easily remember names, numbers, and other important information— maybe even your password! Then we'll give you opportunities to practice your new memory skills.

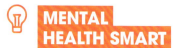 **MENTAL HEALTH SMART**

Don't overlook the role of stress reduction, sleep, and other influences on your mental health. Stress causes your body to release cortisol, and cortisol has been found to shrink the memory centers in the brain, which results in impaired memory.

Meditation has also been proven to substantially improve memory, as has quality sleep. Good, restful sleep is non-negotiable when it comes to thinking fast on your feet. As you transition from slow-wave sleep in the first part of your night to REM sleep in the early morning hours, your memories transform the material you learned throughout the day into actual working knowledge. If you're sleep-deprived, your brain won't retain or recall information as well as it normally would.

Brain health can also be compromised by loneliness, so we've also included plenty of ideas to help you expand your social circle.

 BODY SMART

Piles of research link exercise to stronger memory. Physical activity bathes neural tissue in oxygen-rich blood, increasing the production of brain chemicals that improve memory, attention, and problem-solving skills. Doing more cardio exercise can make your brain actually grow, with more white matter and more neuron connections.

In addition to giving you simple, brain-boosting movement ideas, we'll suggest a few systems checks to ensure your body is helping—not hurting—your brain's capabilities. For example, did you know that blood pressure, hormones, oral health, and medications are associated with your brain's abilities?

Ready to start your best brain-boosting year yet?
All it takes is one day at a time, with small, easy changes to keep your mind sharp. And as you go, we suggest keeping track of favorite hacks, tricks, recipes and tips in the back, on Day 365. Let's go!

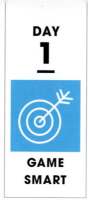

DAY 1 — GAME SMART

Test your creativity with this verbal challenge. **Write a short story.** And we mean *really* short— use just seven words to tell your tale:

DAY 2

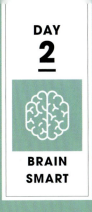

BRAIN SMART

Look in a local newspaper or online entertainment source to find new-to-you museums, great plays, or concerts.

In one study, researchers found that adults over age 50 who made regular trips every few months to cultural attractions—movies, museums, concerts, plays—saw a 32% lower risk of developing depression. Doing this at least once a month bumped that risk reduction up to 48%. **These types of outings combine social interaction, creativity, mental stimulation, and light physical activity, which researchers think all work together to support mental health.** Just as we have a 5-a-day rule for fruit and vegetable consumption, we could also plan regular culture. Where will you go this week?

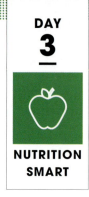

DAY 3 — NUTRITION SMART

Today, familiarize yourself with the MIND diet, and keep track of what you eat in an average day. The MIND diet is based on 10 healthy food groups and 5 not-so-healthy ones. Perfect MIND dieters eat:

- **At least 3 servings** a day of whole grains
- **6 servings** a week of leafy greens, plus **1 serving** a day of one other veggie
- **2 servings** a week of berries
- **1 serving** a week of fish
- **2 servings** a week of poultry
- **3 servings** a week of legumes
- **5 servings** a week of nuts
- **1 serving** a day of alcohol (preferably red wine for its long list of health benefits)

They also use olive oil as the primary oil in their home cooking. As for what they avoid, they nibble on fast or fried foods and cheese less than once a week, and limit their red meat intake to less than 4 times a week. They also keep their sweet tooth in check, eating desserts, pastries or sweets fewer than 5 times a week. Finally, they use less than a tablespoon of butter or margarine a day.

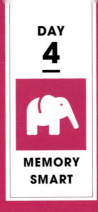

DAY 4

MEMORY SMART

Try the Resize It strategy.

```
      529
    25186
  4295014
 317492706
1528469537
```

It's easier to recall several shorter lists of items—such as numbers—than a long string. For example, we tend to remember a phone number by breaking it up into groups of digits.

With the Resize It technique, you break up a longer list of words or numbers into several shorter lists. Try using this technique to remember the lists of numbers at left. To test yourself, write down each number string after you've applied the Resize It strategy. **See how you did.**

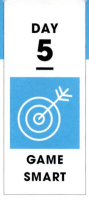

DAY 5

GAME SMART

Remember those connect-the-dots puzzles you did as a kid? See how much of this puzzle you can complete **in 1 minute.** Then erase your work, take a break, and try it again. **Did you get further the second time?**

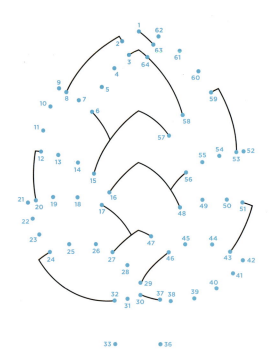

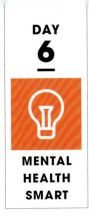

DAY 6 — MENTAL HEALTH SMART

Join a meetup or networking group to expand the circle of people in your life. Plenty of research suggests that broadening your social network and having meaningful relationships is good for your mind. Women with large social networks **slashed their risk of dementia by as much as 26%,** according to one study. Another concluded that maintaining friendships might be the key to a slower decline in memory and cognitive function. Spend 5 to 10 minutes researching potential meetup opportunities, and write them down here:

_____

_____

_____

_____

_____

_____

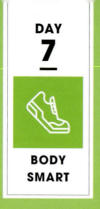

DAY 7

BODY SMART

GO FOR A 10-MINUTE WALK.

Then add 5 minutes each day until your daily walk lasts about 20 minutes. No matter how chaotic your schedule is, you can probably find time for a brief walk every day, and this can pay big dividends in terms of brainpower. Researchers who followed nearly 19,000 women for 2 years and found that those who walked or got some type of moderate exercise for just 90 minutes a week lowered their risk of developing problems with memory and attention span by 20%. **That's less than 13 minutes of exercise a day!**

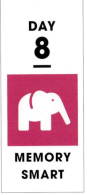

DAY 8

MEMORY SMART

Give your visual attention span a workout.
Study this photograph for 1 minute. Then close the book and write down as many of the items in the photo as you can remember. How did you do?

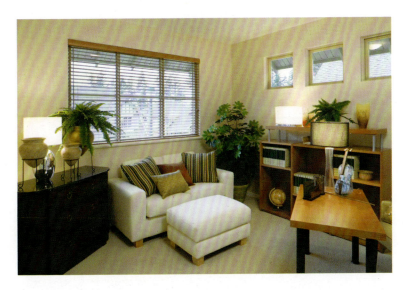

Try a second time, but before you start, take a deep breath and actively focus on the photo. Did you do any better the second time?

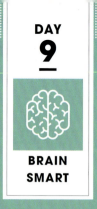

DAY 9

BRAIN SMART

Oops.

Browsing Instagram again? Improve your mental focus by using a digital time management program, such as Time Doctor or RescueTime, to block your access to specific sites. Multitasking makes us feel productive, but that's where it ends. In practice, we're less productive. Our brain is stressed when we multitask, because it wasn't designed to focus on several tasks simultaneously.

What do you need to focus on today?

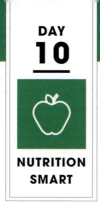

DAY 10

NUTRITION SMART

MAKE A POINT TO DRINK 8 GLASSES OF WATER TODAY.

Every cell in your body needs water to thrive, and your brain cells are no exception. In fact, about 75% of your brain is water, so it's no surprise that getting too little water can result in misery for your mental muscle. Doctors have long known that severe dehydration can cause a person to become confused or disoriented, and (in extreme cases) to slip into a coma. Even mild dehydration may be enough to cause a breakdown in brain functioning, some research suggests. **Chart your water!**

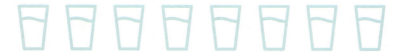

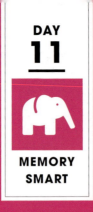

DAY 11
MEMORY SMART

Today, get to know the Rehearse It technique. This strategy requires you to repeat the information you are learning. That's right: You simply restate the information you need to know. Repeat it as many times as you like, either aloud or to yourself. Try it on the same group of numbers you used on Day 4.

5 2 9
2 5 1 8 6
4 2 9 5 0 1 4
3 1 7 4 9 2 7 0 6
1 5 2 8 4 6 9 5 3 7

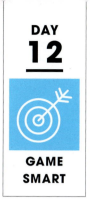

DAY 12

GAME SMART

Word World

Find as many words as you can in 3 minutes in the grid below to bolster pattern recognition and mental processing speed. Words can run in any direction—up, down, sideways, or diagonally—as long as each letter touches the next one. For example, you can form the word BROOM by starting with B, moving left to R, then left again to O, and so on. Try to beat our score of 20.

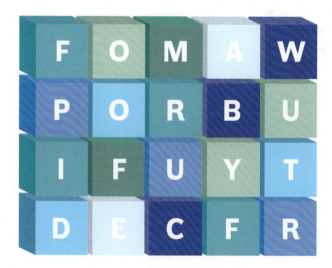

DAY 13

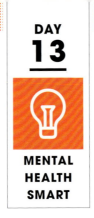

MENTAL HEALTH SMART

DE-STRESS

your future by dealing with things immediately today. Try returning phone calls, paying bills, and answering emails right away, rather than trying to remember to do them days from now.

TODAY

think about which "right now" task could you get done today? Write them down throughout the day.

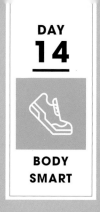

DAY 14

BODY SMART

Don't skip leg day!

Start lifting weights or, if you already lift, learn a new circuit. The boost in cognitive function of older women who did strength training once or twice a week **was nearly 12% higher** than that of women who followed a simple stretching and toning routine. The challenge of learning and mastering different moves can improve brain health.

DAY 15 — GAME SMART

Cryptogram
Can you puzzle out the wisdom here? For solving tips, see Day 190.

_ _ _ _ _ _ N _ O N
1 2 3 4 3 5 6 7 8 5

_ _ _ _ _ _ _ _ _ _
7 9   6 10 3   11 3 9 6

_ _ _ _ _ _ _ _ _
12 3 13 7 14 7 5 3

DAY 16 — BRAIN SMART

On your next work break, visit the watercooler. Researchers found that workers who interacted the most with others had a 34% reduced risk of dementia. In other words, giving your brain some daily exercise in the workplace helps to strengthen networks of connections among brain cells, arming your brain with a more powerful defense against cognitive diseases. If too much solo time at work is a problem, try to team up on projects with colleagues whenever possible.

DAY 17

NUTRITION SMART

Eat 3 servings of vegetables today. One large study showed that veggie lovers are more likely than veggie loathers to maintain brainpower as they age. In fact, people who ate 3 servings of vegetables a day slowed their overall rate of cognitive decline by 40%, compared with those who avoided vegetables, researchers found. How many of these vegetables can you eat this week?

- ☐ Acorn squash
- ☐ Arugula
- ☐ Asparagus
- ☐ Broccoli
- ☐ Brussels sprouts
- ☐ Carrots
- ☐ Cauliflower
- ☐ Celery
- ☐ Cucumber
- ☐ Kale
- ☐ Mushrooms
- ☐ Parsley
- ☐ Potatoes
- ☐ Red bell peppers
- ☐ Romaine lettuce
- ☐ Spinach
- ☐ Sweet potatoes

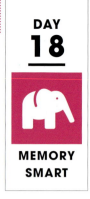

DAY 18
MEMORY SMART

Set your stopwatch for 1 minute and study the photograph below. When the time is up, write down as many objects as you can remember from the photo you just studied.

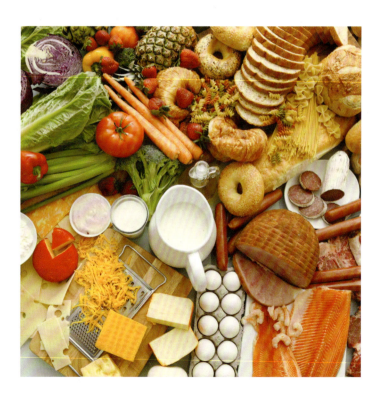

DAY 19 — GAME SMART

Mystery Cube
Which of the options below could be created from the design here?

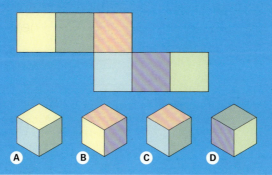

DAY 20 — MENTAL HEALTH SMART

Hug someone!
Your brain grows—even in your later years—in response to pats, hugs, and other physical gestures of affection. Regular socializing also keeps your brain sharp by reducing levels of cortisol, the destructive stress hormone.

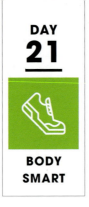

Start an exercise log. Every time you work out, write down in a notebook or journal what you did and how long you did it. Seeing your progress on paper will give your psyche a lift. **Start here:**

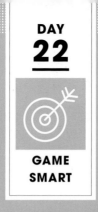

DAY 22

GAME SMART

A limerick

is a humorous, 5-line poem in which the first, second, and fifth lines rhyme with one another and have the same number of syllables (typically 8 or 9). The third and fourth lines are shorter (typically 5 or 6 syllables) and also rhyme with each other. We'll give you the first line: "There once was a gal who was brainy…" Can you finish the limerick?

"There once was a gal who was brainy…"

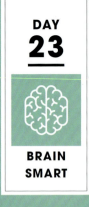

DAY 23

BRAIN SMART

Play a game of chess, checkers, or bridge. All of these games appear to help prevent loss of brain volume (linked to Alzheimer's disease and other forms of dementia), research reveals. This is probably because these types of activities work a variety of areas in your brain, including those that are key for memory, visualization, and sequencing. You could play online, or try an old-fashioned game night with friends—which also might require learning rules, another boost for your brain.

Which game will you try today?

DAY 24

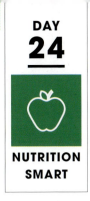

NUTRITION SMART

START

your day right today with a well-rounded breakfast that includes at least 3 food groups. Australian nutritionists who tracked 800 teens found that students scored higher on mental functioning tests with each food group added to their morning meal. A wide range of nutrients may improve the way your brain works, the researchers say. Our ideal morning mix: whole grains + produce + dairy.

- **Whole-grain cereal** with fat-free milk and a small sliced banana

- **Fat-free Greek-style yogurt** with sliced fruit and a handful of rolled oats

- **Whole-grain toast** with low-fat cheese and tomato slices

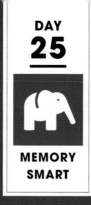

DAY 25

MEMORY SMART

When trying to remember something today, try gazing to your left or right to activate regions of your brain responsible for verbal and spatial memory. Here's what Montclair State research reveals: **Looking left** turns on the parts of your brain responsible for storing spatial information like driving directions. **Gazing right** stokes activity in those brain regions that manage language and speech functions and help you recall things you read or heard.

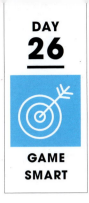

DAY 26
GAME SMART

This brain booster will help hone your visual searching proficiency. This is the skill that helps you spot a friend in a crowded room or even just locate your keys. The table below features many different symbols. Your job is to count the number of times each symbol appears. Here's the catch: You have just 30 seconds per symbol.

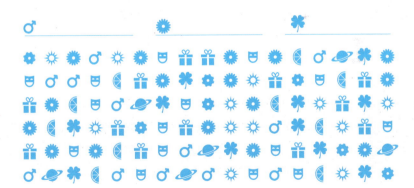

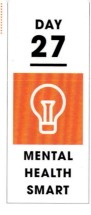

DAY 27 — MENTAL HEALTH SMART

Tonight, turn off all screens before your intended bedtime and read a book instead. Avoid digital screens and TVs for 30 to 60 minutes before bed. The blue light that your devices emit keeps you from producing melatonin, a sleep-supporting hormone that rises in your body at night.

Make a plan:

What time is bedtime? _____

What time will you turn off your TV, phone, tablet, and other digital screens? _____

DAY 28

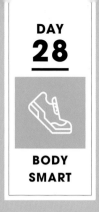

BODY SMART

Today, stand up

when you check your social media feed. If possible, find small ways like this to be active. A large review of studies found that active people have a 35% lower risk of cognitive decline than fitter people. Other research shows that more fit people had stronger brain abilities 25 years later than less-fit types.

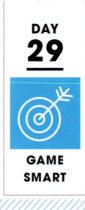

DAY 29 — GAME SMART

Fill in the blanks with the numbers, letters, or symbols that come next in each sequence.

ROW								
1	1	6	11	16	21			
2	4	10	16	22	28			
3	B	D	F	H	J			
4	2	B	4	D	6	F		
5	**	+	\\	*	++	\		

DAY 30

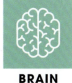

BRAIN SMART

Take a few moments before rising to decide on an intention for your day. Many of us rush through our days on autopilot, going from one errand, family obligation, or social event to another. Researchers have found that we spend up to half of our lives distracted by past or future concerns rather than maintaining full awareness of our surroundings at any given moment. This frenetic activity taxes our brains and our bodies.

This morning, before you do anything else, sit up in bed and focus on the rhythm of your breath for a minute or two. Ask yourself, "What qualities would I like to cultivate today?" If one answer strikes you as especially meaningful, commit yourself to doing your best to stick to that plan for the day, and write it down here:

_____
_____
_____
_____
_____

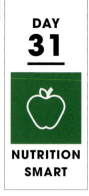

DAY 31
NUTRITION SMART

Most people are pretty good at finding more ways to eat grains or using tricks to fit in their favorite fish, but leafy greens often aren't on the menu. Make eating greens effortless with these strategies:

- **Use Swiss chard** instead of basil in your favorite pesto—just steam or blanch the leaves and work them into the usual recipe, then toss it with pasta or spoon it over salmon.

- **When having poached or fried eggs** for breakfast, skip the toast and serve the eggs over sautéed spinach.

- **Smother a healthy homemade veggie-topped pizza** with arugula.

- **Don't like bitter greens?** Sweeten them up: Roast grapes in olive oil and herbs, then toss handfuls of kale over the grapes and pop the whole thing back into the oven for a moment. Serve over pasta.

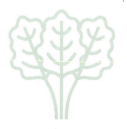

DAY 32

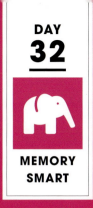

MEMORY SMART

Test yourself using the Label It strategy.

This technique is similar to Resize It, which you learned on Day 4. But it adds an element: Often, some items on a long list are related to one another, making them easy to group into categories. Instead of randomly breaking up entries on a long list, divide them into natural groupings and give each one a label—produce, dry goods, fish, baked goods, and so on. These labels act as hints to help you recall the items on each smaller list.

- ☐ Apples
- ☐ Salt
- ☐ Flour
- ☐ Cod
- ☐ Oatmeal
- ☐ Muffins
- ☐ Bagels
- ☐ Celery
- ☐ Quinoa
- ☐ Trout
- ☐ Shrimp
- ☐ Pears
- ☐ Spinach
- ☐ Biscuits
- ☐ Salmon
- ☐ Cookies

Try using both techniques to memorize the grocery list at left. Read the list of items once, close the book, and write down as many as you can remember. How did you do?

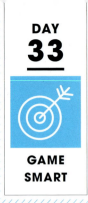

DAY 33 — GAME SMART

Berry Good at Math

What number does each berry represent?

🍓 + 🍓 + 🍓 = 15

🍓 + 🫐 + 🫐 = 19

🍓 + 🫐 + 🍇 = 21

🫐 + 🍇 + 🫐 = 23

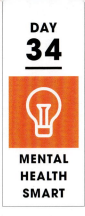

DAY 34

MENTAL HEALTH SMART

Take up knitting or another needlecraft such as embroidery, quilting, crochet, or macrame. Chain craft stores and local mom-and-pop shops offer in-store knitting classes that range from basic to more specialized. Repetitive motions used in knitting and other needlecrafts can be soothing and elicit your body's relaxation response—the same calm, meditative feeling some people get from formal mindfulness practices or yoga.

A survey of more than 3,500 knitters found that 81% of those who suffered from depression described feeling happier and calmer after clicking their needles. Other studies have shown that knitting can curb rumination (repetitive negative thoughts) in people with eating disorders, lessen the focus on chronic pain, and provide a respite from depressive thoughts.

Look up locations where you can get your knit on, and write them down here:

_____
_____
_____
_____

DAY 35

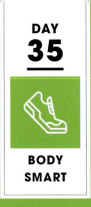

BODY SMART

Go for a swim. Among older women, aerobic exercise—including joint-friendly swimming—significantly increased the volume of the brain's hippocampus. This is the structure involved in verbal memory and learning. The more you move, the more oxygen- and nutrient-carrying blood flows to and nourishes your brain, the study authors say. If you want a healthy memory, you need to exercise.

What aerobic exercise did you do today?

_____
_____
_____
_____
_____

DAY 36 **GAME SMART**

Solve the following brainteaser. What are the next 3 letters in the following sequence?

J   F

M   A   M   J

J   A   ☐   ☐   ☐

DAY 37 **BRAIN SMART**

Today, stay clear and focused by setting your thermostat to the low 70s. Feeling cold can be so distracting that it impairs your thinking. One study found that increasing office temperatures by 9°F led to a 44% reduction in typing errors. But being too warm also hampers performance: In other research, temperatures higher than 75°F were linked to decreased productivity.

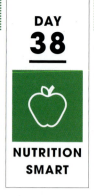

DAY 38 — NUTRITION SMART

This morning, don't skip your protein. In one experiment, researchers gave 22 people a high-protein, low-carb breakfast, and then a low-protein, high-carb meal a week later. After each meal, the participants played a game: One player proposed a way to divide a sum of money; if the other player rejected it, no one got the cash. Those who ate the high-protein breakfast were more likely to accept unreasonable offers. Researchers believe the protein-laden meal created higher levels of the amino acid tyrosine—part of the brain's "reward system"—which may have made players feel more satisfied with less.

What protein source did you have at breakfast this morning?

_____
_____
_____

DAY 39

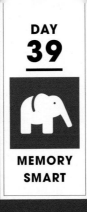

MEMORY SMART

Sharpen your ability to remember new information with the Relate It hack. With this strategy, the idea is to associate, or "link," new information that you're learning with a familiar concept. A link can be the name of a friend or other acquaintance, a celebrity or famous historical figure, or an object that you connect with the name.

Or you might link a string of numbers you need to remember to a date on the calendar.

In that way, the string 1 0 2 4 would become October 24.

Try it with the numbers you learned earlier on Day 4.

DAY 40 — GAME SMART

Math Square
Put a different number between 1 and 9 in each box to make all the equations correct.

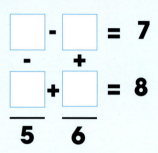

DAY 41 — MENTAL HEALTH SMART

Pick up an adult coloring book and some colored pencils (or just a pen and piece of paper), and scribble and shade your way to zen. Coloring can be a simple way to de-stress before bed, especially. In fact, research shows that this simple pastime has therapeutic benefits. Art therapy, which includes coloring, can help with depression, anxiety, and post-traumatic stress disorder, or PTSD.

DAY 42 **BODY SMART**

Block out time in your schedule for a workout. If you write down "20-minute walk" in the space for noon in your day planner, treat the walk like an appointment that you can't miss or reschedule. What time will you exercise today?

DAY 43 **GAME SMART**

Middleman

For each pair, find a word that creates two new compound words or phrases. It should work as the ending of the first word and the beginning of the second.

CORK	ROOM
SUN	HOUSE
LIFE	LINE
PINE	SAUCE
TAKE	SIDE

DAY 44

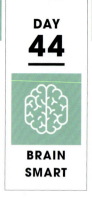

BRAIN SMART

Today at lunchtime, spend 5 to 10 minutes intentionally daydreaming. Several recent experiments have found that letting your mind wander may help your brain to better catalog and store memories. One study in the journal *Neuron* suggests that daydreaming helps improve your memory in ways similar to sleeping or napping.

At what time did you daydream? _____

What did you think about?

_____
_____
_____
_____
_____

DAY 45

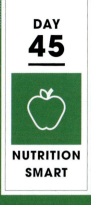

NUTRITION SMART

Caffeine

is a stimulant, so it fights off fatigue and increases alertness. In the lab, tests show that caffeine improves attention span, reaction time, and other brain skills. But experts recommend limiting yourself to 300–400 milligrams of caffeine a day, tops. More can lead to insomnia.

Use this chart to select your beverage boost without undermining your brain's beauty sleep.

	Caffeine (milligrams)
Dark chocolate 1 oz	5 to 35
Iced tea 8 oz	9 to 50
Brewed tea 8 oz	20 to 90
Cola 12 oz	30
Espresso 1 shot	58 to 76
Brewed coffee 8 oz	72 to 130
Red Bull® energy drink 8 oz	80

DAY 46

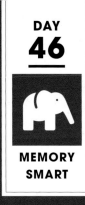

MEMORY SMART

Skip googling. The next time you can't remember an actor's name, don't reach for your phone. Tech tools fuel a modern-day condition called digital amnesia—forgetting information because you trust a computerized device to remember it for you.

When you learn new information and then recall it later, you activate 2 brain areas intimately involved with memory—the hippocampus and the prefrontal cortex. But when you rely on external memory joggers, such as your phone or the Internet, those brain regions can weaken. The next time you find yourself struggling to name a celebrity, challenge yourself to not look it up.

What did you skip googling, and remember today?

_____
_____
_____

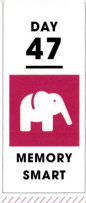

DAY 47

MEMORY SMART

Crack the Code

Which set of letters describes the picture in the final box?

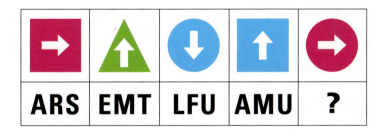

A: AFT   **B:** ERS   **C:** ALU   **D:** LRS

BONUS: Can you rearrange the 12 letters in this puzzle into a word that describes your puzzling skills?

DAY 48

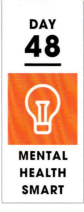

MENTAL HEALTH SMART

Consider taking a community dance class. Whether it's flamenco or foxtrot, dancing can boost your mood and lower your stress and anxiety. What's more, it'll improve your balance and flexibility and could even improve your heart health. Researchers using MRI scans found that in addition to better balance, older adults who took weekly choreographed dance classes saw an increase in the size of their hippocampus, a part of the brain that plays a significant role in memory and learning. And joining a group can boost your sense of belonging, also a mental health positive. **Write down some classes you could take.**

_____

_____

_____

_____

_____

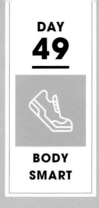

DAY 49

BODY SMART

Today, practice juggling for 5 minutes with either 3 small balls or scarves. Start out with one small ball, slowly tossing it in the air from one hand to the other to form a big loop. When you've mastered one ball, add another. Now try 3. Don't worry if you find it too hard; switch to juggling scarves, which are easier to grab and fall more gracefully. Having fun? Keep at it: A recent study suggests that juggling might help build brain volume. That could mean an increase in new connections between synapses and a more robust cognitive reserve.

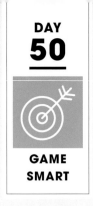

DAY 50

GAME SMART

Rebus Rally: Each of the word combinations below represents a common phrase.
Can you figure out all 10? To get you started, we'll give you the first one: "Big bad wolf."
Can you see why?

1. **BAD** wolf

2. S
   L
   O
   W

3. R | E | A | D

4. Thought Clever

5. M
   R
   A
   W

6. EGGS
   EASY

7. TOUKEEPCH

8. NOON GOOD

9. T
   A
   BLE

10. EVIL
    --------> evil

DAY 51

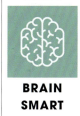

BRAIN SMART

If your mind often wanders during work or Zoom meetings, try the following:

Eliminate distractions. If you have several to-do's, pick one to tackle first, and clear all other projects off your desk and computer screen.

Participate. If you daydream during meetings, challenge yourself by thinking of questions to ask, and raise your hand as much as possible. You may miss a moment if you're formulating a question, but you'll stay focused on the current topic.

Take a break. When your concentration starts to slip during the workday, leave your desk and take a walk outside or to the office common space for a mental breather. This way, your brain associates your desk only with work, not mind wandering.

After all, if you don't take regular breaks—especially when you're not enjoying your job—your brain will take them for you.

Which strategy worked best for you?

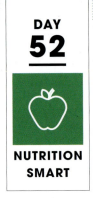

DAY 52 — NUTRITION SMART

Minimize your mercury intake from seafood. Mercury affects not only cognition—clear thinking—but also (and especially) the cerebellum. That's the part of your brain that controls balance, coordination, and vision. Want to reduce your exposure to mercury found in fish? Follow this advice from the Environmental Protection Agency:

1. Do not eat shark, swordfish, king mackerel, or tilefish; these species contain high levels of mercury.

2. Eat up to 12 oz (2 average meals) a week of a lower-mercury variety of fish or shellfish, such as shrimp, canned light tuna, salmon, pollock, and catfish.

3. When choosing your 2 meals of fish or shellfish, limit white (albacore) tuna to 6 ounces a week.

DAY 53

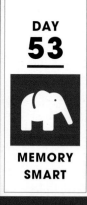

MEMORY SMART

The See It strategy requires you to visualize, or "see" in your mind, the information you are trying to learn. The more vivid and detailed the image, the better this technique will work for you.
Try it with the word list below:

GAME	EGG	HONOR
PEN	BENCH	STRIPE
WELT	FAN	PHONE

DAY 54 GAME SMART

Word Sequence Which of these choices should come next in the sentence? (Hint: Consider the characteristics of the words.)

A BOY COULD DELIGHT _____

A. EVERYBODY   **B.** NOBODY   **C.** EVERYONE

DAY 55 GAME SMART

Using the following cipher, decode the message below.

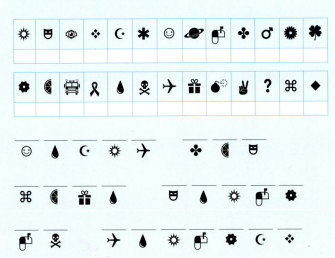

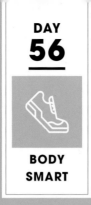

DAY 56
BODY SMART

Get extra exercise today. A 30-minute cardio workout is great for burning calories and boosting the production of essential brain chemicals. But if you push yourself to go for 45 minutes, those benefits increase by 50%. Today, sneak in a little extra exercise on top of your normal workouts. For example, instead of meeting a friend for drinks or dinner, invite your pal to go for a walk—or at least meet early and take a walk before dinner.

How will you get extra exercise today?

_____
_____
_____

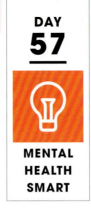

DAY 57 — MENTAL HEALTH SMART

Try revising your negative mental statements today. Reframing negative self-talk (catastrophizing, self-blame, blaming others, and defeatist thinking) is one technique you can use to set yourself on a positive path.

Instead of: "I never get the best assignments at work. My boss must think I'm an idiot."

Try: "My boss doesn't yet know what I'm capable of. I'll come up with a list of new projects I'd love to tackle, and that will help her see me in a new light."

Instead of: "I brought this breakup on myself—I always pick losers who can't commit."

Try: "Blaming myself or my ex won't make me feel better. What did I learn from this relationship that will help me find a more compatible partner next time?"

What's one statement you often catch yourself thinking about?

___

___

How can you reframe and rephrase?

___

___

DAY 58

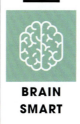

BRAIN SMART

If you can't always find the right word, relax:

Not all memory lapses spell trouble. These examples may help you distinguish normal age-related memory glitches from dementia.

Don't worry

- Being unable to recall the details of a conversation or event of a year ago
- Occasionally forgetting appointments or names
- Sometimes searching for the right word
- Fretting about your memory when no one else is, including your family

Talk with your doctor

- Being unable to recall the details of an event or conversation that happened last week
- Forgetting things you once remembered easily
- Frequently pausing to find the right word, or using substitute words when the right one won't come to mind
- Not worrying about your memory, while relatives or friends are expressing concern

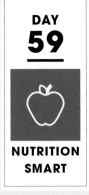

DAY 59

NUTRITION SMART

Sugar

by any other name is still too sweet. Any type of sugar that's added to food during preparation or processing can cause issues. That includes agave, corn sweeteners, honey, and more. People with blood sugar levels at the high end of the normal range were more likely to lose brain volume in the hippocampus and amygdala (areas involved in memory and cognition) than were people who had lower blood sugar levels, an Australian study found. Added sugars may take the form of:

	Sucrose
	Evaporated cane juice
	Agave nectar
	Fruit juice concentrate
	100% fruit juice
	High-fructose corn syrup
	Galactose, maltose, dextrose, lactose, and other "ose" additives
	Blackstrap molasses
	Organic brown rice syrup

How many did you find in your pantry?
Place a check mark to the left of each sugar.

DAY 60

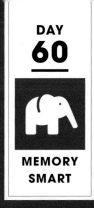

MEMORY SMART

Who doesn't love a good story?

You can make a list more memorable by turning it into a fun, creative story using the Tales technique. The stranger and more outlandish, the better. It'll be attention-grabbing and meaningful, making you more likely to remember the information. **Try memorizing the word list below with Tales.**

BOY	METHOD
PADDOCK	JUMP
TOWER	VINE
CLUB	STEAM
WIND	DECK

Give your visual speed a workout with this a-maze-ing task.

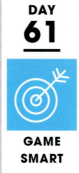

DAY 61

GAME SMART

Using a pencil, trace your way through the maze below.

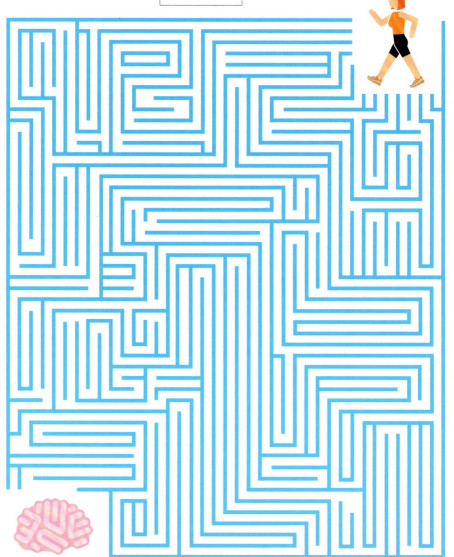

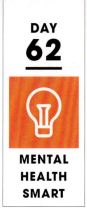

DAY 62 — MENTAL HEALTH SMART

Grow some gratitude. Write down 3 to 5 things you're grateful for today. To get the most out of this practice, don't just dash off a laundry list. Instead, stop and contemplate why you feel grateful, being as specific as possible: *I'm grateful for my new neighbor, who helped me dig out my car in the freezing cold.* Or *I've been worried about Dad, so I'm glad he was feeling up to talking to me on the phone.*

In one study, people who wrote 5 sentences about a single positive thing got more of a boost than those who wrote 1 sentence about each of 5 different things.

_____
_____
_____
_____

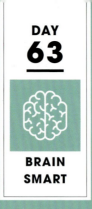

DAY 63

BRAIN SMART

Build new neuronal connections by putting your nondominant hand into action. Use the hand that you don't usually use to perform such daily tasks as brushing your teeth, combing your hair, applying makeup (careful with mascara!), eating, and so on. Try writing with your other hand too. **Does using your nondominant hand get any easier as the day proceeds?**

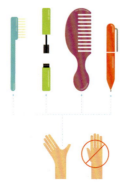

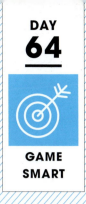

DAY 64

GAME SMART

Word World

Find as many words as you can in this letter grid in 3 minutes. Words can run in any direction—up, down, sideways, or diagonally—as long as each letter adjoins the following letter. For example, you can form the word LARGE by starting with L, moving up to A, diagonally to R, and so on.

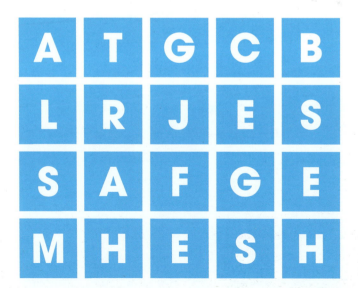

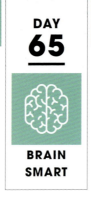

DAY 65

BRAIN SMART

Download and listen to a classical music playlist today, or just turn on a classical radio station. In a study published in the journal *Scientific Reports*, University of Helsinki scientists found that listening to classical music can boost brainpower at any age. By affecting dopamine pathways, music may silence the genes that are risk factors for dementia.

Write down any favorite playlists you come across today.

_____
_____
_____
_____
_____
_____

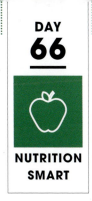

DAY 66 — NUTRITION SMART

Cook a MIND dish today, which is healthy for your brain in 2 ways. Cooking requires a variety of mental functions: organization (gathering ingredients); problem solving (finding a substitute for that missing clove of garlic); hand-eye coordination (chopping and mincing things); and multitasking and concentration (rushing from the stove to the oven to the fridge).

What's more, cooking uses 4 of your 5 senses—smell, touch, sight, and taste—which all utilize different parts of your brain.

Whole-Grain Tabbouleh Salad

INGREDIENTS

- 1 cup cooked quinoa, millet, or barley
- 1¾ cup vegetable broth
- 1 large ripe tomato, diced
- ½ cup finely chopped cucumber
- ⅓ cup chopped scallions
- ⅓ cup chopped fresh mint
- ¼ cup chopped fresh parsley and tender stems
- ¼ cup extra virgin olive oil
- 3 Tbsp fresh lemon juice

1. **Cook quinoa** (or other grain) with vegetable broth per package directions.

2. **Spread quinoa** onto a sheet pan to cool. (If you prepare your quinoa a day in advance, you can skip this step and refrigerate it until ready to use.) Transfer cool quinoa to a salad or mixing bowl.

3. **Add** tomato, cucumber, scallions, mint, parsley, oil, lemon juice, and salt and pepper to taste. Stir well. Cover and chill before serving.

DAY 67

MEMORY SMART

The Videos technique

is simply the YouTube version of Tales. (See Day 60.) Use items on a list to create a short movie in your mind. Again, putting the items into an offbeat, funny, or bizarre story will make them more memorable.

••

Try memorizing this word list used earlier, this time with the Videos approach.

BOY	METHOD
PADDOCK	JUMP
TOWER	VINE
CLUB	STEAM
WIND	DECK

DAY 68

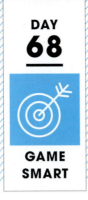

GAME SMART

Cryptogram

Crack the code to find some advice from Eleanor Roosevelt. For solving tips, see Day 190.

```
  Y              T           T
- --- ---    - --- --- ---  -- ---  --- ---
 MAI BIJH     LA HSD
```

```
  T              Y
- --- --- --- ---   --- --- ---
 HSFWX        MAI
```

```
  T              Y
- --- --- --- ---   --- --- ---
 HSFWU        MAI
```

```
       T
- --- --- --- ---   -- ---
 RZWWAH       LA
```

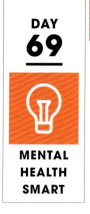

DAY 69

MENTAL HEALTH SMART

Today, grab binoculars (or your eagle eyes) to go watch some birds. You can head out solo to a forest preserve or connect with other locals. Find birding buddies through the National Audubon Society (audubon.org) or the nonprofit American Birding Association (aba.org). There's a mountain of evidence confirming the magic of spending time outdoors: lower cortisol levels and blood pressure, better mood and concentration, and a greater sense of relaxation and calm. If you don't have time to join a group, just set up a feeder: One study found that the more birds people spotted from their windows, the lower their levels of anxiety and depression, whether or not they were able to identify the species.

Name 3 birds you saw today. If you don't know the names, just describe the feathered friends:

_____
_____
_____

DAY 70

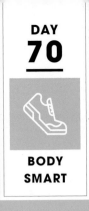

BODY SMART

Find a workout buddy. Having a partner can help on those days when you don't feel like exercising. In one study, researchers found that women trying to lose weight were more likely to succeed if they joined a support group than if they worked out alone in a gym. **List a few people you could ask to work up a sweat with:**

_____

_____

_____

_____

_____

_____

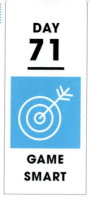

Missing Piece
Which shape will fit in the space?

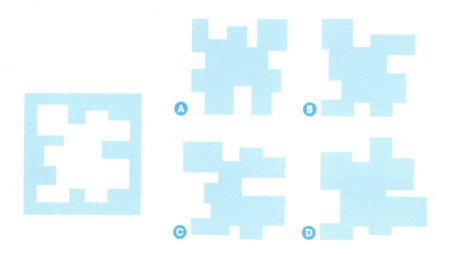

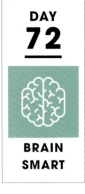

DAY 72

BRAIN SMART

Today, practice these Attention ER techniques when you lose focus. The trick is knowing how to get it back. Try each a few times, then pick one that you can turn to the next time you need laser-sharp focus:

- **Count** backward from 20.
- **Take** several slow, deep breaths.
- **Breathe** into your heart: Think of an image that makes you feel safe and happy—yourself sitting on a beach, perhaps, or the face of a loved one. Now take several slow, deep breaths, as if you're trying to fill your heart with air each time you inhale.

Which technique worked best?

_____

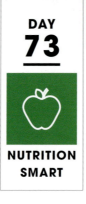

DAY 73

NUTRITION SMART

Make a spinach dip. Popeye only gobbled spinach greens for his guns, but in one study, eating a single serving of spinach a day was associated with a slowing of cognitive decline in older adults. Credit goes to its vitamin K, folate, beta-carotene, and lutein. Not into spinach? Kale, broccoli, chard, and collard greens all boast a similar makeup of nutrients.

Zesty Spinach Dip: Blend a cup of baby spinach with a 6 oz container of plain Greek yogurt, some chopped scallions, salt, and the juice of half a lime. Scoop it up with more veggies—a double dose to help keep your brain sharp.

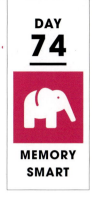

DAY 74

MEMORY SMART

Creating an alliteration—a phrase that uses repeating consonant sounds, can help boost your memory, studies have found. In one study, people read poetry and prose both quietly and aloud. Later, they were able to recall passages containing alliterative phrases much better than others. Keep the phrases simple: "Dial the doctor," "last laugh," "sink or swim."

Can you think of alliterative fits for these common to-do list entries?

Keep keys in the _____

Bake _____

Pick up _____

Call _____

Now create a few of your own: _____

_____

_____

_____

| DAY **75** | | GAME SMART |

Phrase Anagrams

Rearrange the letters in each of these phrases to create a new, related phrase.

THE EYES
_ _ _ _   _ _ _

ELEVEN PLUS TWO
_ _ _ _ _ _   _ _ _ _   _ _ _

CERTAINLY NOT
_ _ _ _ ,   _ _ _ _   _ _   _ _

| DAY **76** | | MENTAL HEALTH SMART |

Today, try meditating for 5 minutes using an app like Calm, or stream a guided session via Spotify. Meditation may even make you smarter. Researchers note that people who've meditated for 4 years or longer have a higher degree of something called gyrification, which is crucial for memory and consciousness.

DAY 77

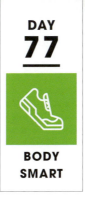

BODY SMART

Who needs a fancy indoor bike? Not you. Today, try a 10- to 30-minute no-frills rhythm workout to upbeat music. Here are the cool moves:

- **March in place:** Pump your arms, keeping them close to your body, as if you're power walking. Be sure to land softly on your feet and try to keep your arms moving.

- **Jumping jacks**

- **Jog:** Try to keep in time with the music.

- **Pushups:** Try to keep in time with the music.

- **High knees:** Bring your knees up as high as you can. Pump your arms for more intensity.

- **Step-ups:** Use a stair and step your right foot up first, followed by the left. Then step your right foot back down, then left. Keep alternating feet. Use your arms to drive yourself up.

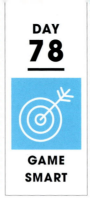

DAY 78

GAME SMART

Word World

In 3 minutes, find as many words as you can in the grid below to bolster pattern recognition and mental processing speed. Words can run in any direction—up, down, sideways, or diagonally—as long as each letter touches the next one. For example, you can form the word KITE by starting with K, moving up to I, and so on. Try to beat our score of 16.

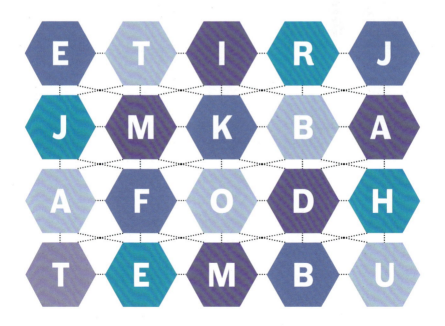

DAY 79

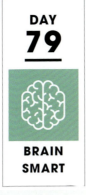

BRAIN SMART

LET'S TALK DIRTY

No, not that kind of dirty. Science shows that the benefits of gardening include greater life satisfaction, less fatigue, and a 36% lower risk of dementia for people who garden daily. Botanical gardens and arboretums in your area may host gardening workshops and classes. If you don't have space for a garden in your backyard, check out the American Community Gardening Association's website (communitygarden.org) to find a plot near your home.

Community gardens can boost social ties and a sense of neighborly unity, research suggests. Plus, being outdoors digging around just feels good.

DAY 80 **NUTRITION SMART**

Add some beans to your diet today.
Homemade black bean soup and pinto bean chili are delicious, but if you're not a cook, just throw some chickpeas on a salad. Beans are packed with fiber, which research links to enhanced cognition. Aim for at least 3 servings a week; one serving equals ½ cup cooked beans.

DAY 81 **GAME SMART**

RIDDLE: I have keys but no keyholes. What am I?

DAY 82

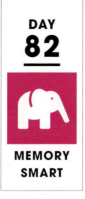

MEMORY SMART

Today, test out the Domino technique.

Sometimes remembering all the items on a list isn't enough—you need to know them in order. For example, say you need to memorize the key talking points for a speech or presentation at work. Or you need to recall a set of directions. The Domino technique lets the information fall into place.

To use this technique, mentally connect one item on the list with the subsequent item by creating a visual scenario. For example, if calendar, gloves, shoelaces, and plate are listed, you could connect the *calendar* to the *gloves* by imagining a calendar illustrated with gloves. To link gloves to *shoelaces*, picture a pair of gloved hands tying a shoe. To connect the last 2 words, visualize the shoelaces being placed on a *plate*.

Use the Domino technique to remember the list of words below.

HUT	**FOOT**	**CANDY**
CANDLE	**POUR**	**SANDAL**
RECORD	**BRUSH**	**GOOSE**

DAY 83

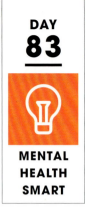

MENTAL HEALTH SMART

To lift the blues in minutes, turn your thoughts into a race. For example, when your mother-in-law is driving you crazy, give yourself 30 seconds to make a list of all the ways she's been helpful to you in the past. You'll feel better fast. If nothing nice comes to mind, quickly jot down other ways she bugs you. Really: Speed-thinking negative thoughts can still improve your mood. Researchers believe that rapid thinking may release feel-good brain chemicals. **Or it could just be a helpful distraction.**

DAY 84

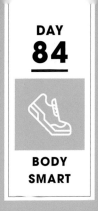

BODY SMART

Take a balance test.

Practice standing on one leg, with the other leg raised and eyes open for up to 60 seconds. Balance is achieved and maintained by 3 main sensory circuits: Vision, proprioception (your sense of body position), and the vestibular system (your inner ear). If you can't keep your balance past 20 seconds after a few tries, then you may be at increased risk for brain disease and cognitive decline. **Talk to your health care provider.**

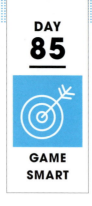

DAY 85

GAME SMART

Everyone has some artistic skill, even if it's hidden. Find yours by forcing your brain to think in a totally new way. Draw a portrait of yourself. **The catch: Your pen can touch the paper only 5 times.**

DAY 86

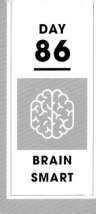

BRAIN SMART

Find a funny TikTok, *SNL* skit, or TV show. Stress and its repercussions (inflammation, poor sleep) have been shown to mess with your memory. Laughter not only counteracts stress but also improves your short-term memory, according to a series of research efforts. In fact, just 20 minutes of watching a funny video can be enough to bolster short-term memory, research reveals.

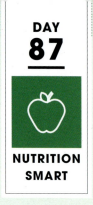

DAY 87

NUTRITION SMART

Before making any decisions today, fuel up on a healthy snack. An empty stomach can make you more impulsive, one study found. When you've consumed enough calories, you can focus on the outcome of a tough choice instead of being distracted by immediate needs—like food for survival.

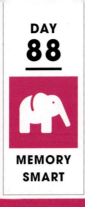

DAY 88

MEMORY SMART

Use one of the memory techniques from the past few weeks to memorize words you need to recall. Jot down some information you want to remember (such as a set of directions) on the worksheet below. Now commit it to memory by practicing your newly honed strategy for learning words.

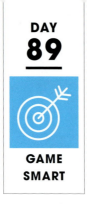

DAY 89

GAME SMART

Here's a brain challenge that will help you discover the artist within. Using the space below, draw as many objects as you can using three straight lines of the same length.

DAY 90

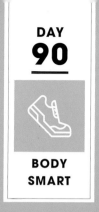

BODY SMART

Try *qigong*.

If you're afflicted by midday brain drain, sometimes movement, not rest, is just the thing to give you a jolt. *Qigong* is an ancient Chinese practice designed to enhance the flow of *qi*, or energy. It's a series of gentle movements that are synchronized with your breathing.

There are many styles and routines, but one quick *qigong* energy exercise is called Flying Like an Eagle: Stand with feet parallel and shoulder-width apart, knees slightly bent, arms at your sides, and fingers slightly apart and curved. Breathe in and rise up on your toes, bringing your arms up and out until your hands are at ear height. Breathe out as you slowly lower your heels and bring your arms down to your thighs. **Do in one fluid motion for 10 reps.**

DAY 91 BRAIN SMART

If you take the same route to work or the gym every day, get out a map and plan a new one. Want to give your mind a greater challenge? Forget the map and find your own way.

If you "remapped" your brain today, where did you go?

DAY 92 GAME SMART

Anyone can read backward. But understanding what you read requires some well-toned mental muscles. Give yours a flex: Choose an article in today's newspaper and read it backward, beginning with the last word in the story and working your way to the first. Can you make sense of what you read? If you don't have a newspaper handy, try reading Day 102 aloud.

DAY 93

BRAIN SMART

Take up sewing, sculpting, woodworking, or painting. Engaging in creative hobbies can reduce your risk of developing mild cognitive impairment by anywhere from 45% to 73%, according to one study. If you don't have the time or desire to take a class, try to set aside a few hours each week to do something crafty. Don't know where to start? You can find DIY kits on Etsy. Write down a hobby you think you might not be "creative" enough to do, and then find a class for beginners. **You might be surprised. Or pick up an easy kit, even if it's just a paint-by-number.**

_____
_____
_____
_____
_____

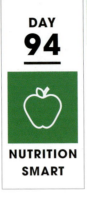

DAY 94 — NUTRITION SMART

Check your diet for vitamin D today.

Research links vitamin D to all sorts of health benefits, and several studies draw connections between this "sunshine vitamin" and both brain health and memory. One associated higher vitamin D levels with improved verbal memory scores. Another study, this one from the U.K., hinted that vitamin D might have a protective effect against dementia. You can pick up vitamin D in fortified milk and fatty fish.

Which foods are you getting your vitamin D from today?

_____

_____

_____

_____

_____

DAY 95

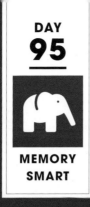

MEMORY SMART

Today you'll sing

for your synapses with a brain stretch that lets you show off your musical side. Create a jingle by putting the following words to music. Don't worry, this isn't a contest. **The goal is simply to get in the groove and challenge your brain.**

HEART	DANDELION
BOX	PUFF
MATTER	HAIR
SUGAR	FOREST
RAW	

DAY 96

GAME SMART

Think fast: How well do you know your multiplication tables? Beginning with 0 x 0, see how far you can get in 3 minutes. (Stop if you reach 12 x 12.) Repeat 3 times and time yourself.

How far did you get?

_____

Try again. How far did you get this time?

_____

Experiment with this: Try it again at another time of day. Does stress or fatigue impact your speed?

_____

_____

DAY 97

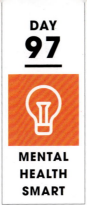

MENTAL HEALTH SMART

The next time something threatens to stress you out, take a step back and view things from an outside perspective instead of panicking about what it may mean for the future. If it were happening to a friend, what would you advise your friend to do? Being an observer keeps you in a calm, slightly detached place. This helps you become more solution-oriented.

If there's something that happens today that causes you worry, write it here:

_____
_____
_____
_____

DAY 98

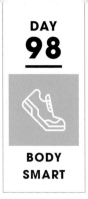

BODY SMART

Take a nature walk without headphones, in a park if possible. Researchers found that memory and attention improved 20% when people walked in a park versus an urban environment. Busy surroundings—noisy traffic, colorful billboards, throngs of people—are distracting and clamor for your attention. Music can have the same effect, so leave your device at home. You'll emerge calmer, more focused, and better able to tackle your to-do list.

Where did you go?

_____

_____

Where will you walk next?

_____

_____

DAY 99 **GAME SMART**

List It
Boost your recall power by writing down as many dog breeds as you can think of in 1 minute. We got 15. **How did you do?**

DAY 100 **GAME SMART**

Puzzle
Which puzzle piece will fit in the empty spot?

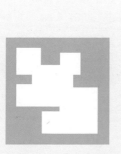
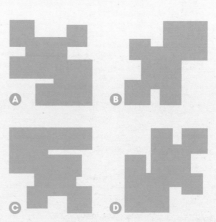

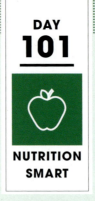

DAY 101

NUTRITION SMART

Make your own trail mix for today's snack: Choose various nuts (cashews, hazelnuts, almonds, walnuts) and dried or freeze-dried berries (blueberries, strawberries, or raspberries). A recent review suggests that nuts and berries may help boost memory and fight depression. The bonuses were most evident in older adults. That's good news in the fight against cognitive aging.

Try to eat ½ cup of nuts and 1 to 2 cups of berries a day. Fresh or frozen are best, but dried berries (about ½ to 1 cup) are good, too.

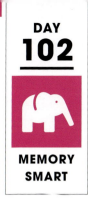

DAY 102 — MEMORY SMART

Grab a pen and paper and read the following paragraph. When you finish reading, set your stopwatch for 2 minutes and write down as much of the story as you remember. Include all the details you can recall, in any order. No peeking! Rely only on your memory. Stop when the 2 minutes are up.

When the 2 minutes are up, stop and close the book. Ethan Brown and his wife, Emma, plan to open a children's shoe store. They looked for a location near the center of town in Clarkston. They first saw a basement-level site on Oak Street, but it was too dark. On Thursday, they found a place on Mission Street. It is at street level, with large windows facing the sidewalk. It has a storage area in the rear. There is a playground across the street that is always filled with parents and small children. After signing the lease, Ethan and Emma went to their favorite restaurant, Jimmy's, to celebrate and eat lunch. Emma, who had worked for 13 years at a store called If the Shoe Fits in the nearby city of Hartsville, decided to have a play area in the front of the store with a large bin for dress-up clothes. They'll name their store Brown's Shoes.

DAY 103

BRAIN SMART

Pick up some great reads. Men and women who frequently spent time reading, playing board games, or playing musical instruments had a significantly reduced risk of dementia, one study found. Get book recommendations from coworkers, Facebook friends—and the best source of all, your local librarian. **Write them below:**

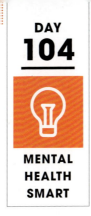

DAY 104 — MENTAL HEALTH SMART

Try this mindfulness exercise. Adapted from the work of Jon Kabat-Zinn, Ph.D., mindfulness teaches you how to use all of your senses to experience more every day.

When was the last time you really thought about...a raisin? Grab a raisin and, instead of popping it into your mouth, spend time observing its appearance. How does it feel in your hand? How would you describe its aroma? Now put it in your mouth and chew slowly. What sensations do you experience? Write your impressions below.

_____

_____

_____

_____

_____

_____

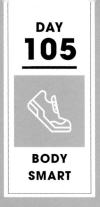

DAY 105

BODY SMART

Do a 7-minute workout.

You don't need fancy equipment or even a lot of time to squeeze in a great workout. Just go outside and find something sturdy to step up on, like a bench. Then do 7 minutes' worth of exercise. Yes, that's it! Scientists have found that this amount of intense exercise can do as much good as a more extended cardio session plus a workout with weights. Check out the Johnson & Johnson Official 7 Minute Workout app for some new moves. **Aim for 7 to 12 exercises; do each for 30 seconds, and then rest for 10 seconds before the next one.**

DAY 106 GAME SMART

Resale Riddle
A woman buys an antique lamp for $40, then sells it for $50. Later, she buys it back for $60, spends $5 fixing it up, and sells it again for $75.
Did she make any money, and if so, how much?

DAY 107 MEMORY SMART

Here's a useful memory hack: Tracking down information you infrequently use can be challenging, so try storing it in a Memory Log. A small address book works well for this purpose. For example, if you want to keep track of where you keep your will, turn to the W page, jot down "will," and note the will's location.

DAY 108

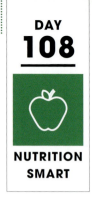

NUTRITION SMART

Here's a great way to get great brain-enhancing nutrients right from the get-go: Steel-cut oats with blueberries, strawberries, and a dash of cinnamon. Enjoy with a cup of coffee.

The whole-grain foundation of this morning meal is based on the MIND diet, which calls for at least 3 servings of whole grains a day. Topping those great grains with blueberries and strawberries adds extra oomph to this breakfast's brain benefits. According to research:

- **The flavonoids found in berries** significantly slow cognitive decline.

- **Adding a sprinkle of cinnamon** not only perks up your senses, but also boosts your memory.

- **Last but not least: coffee.** Research finds caffeine intake (paired with a healthy diet) benefits cognition and may also slow age-related declines in memory and attention span.

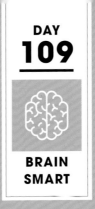

DAY 109

BRAIN SMART

When you notice a

BEAUTIFUL

tree, or some wildflowers at the farmers' market, post a photo. Taking a photo a day and putting it on social media has a number of benefits that can boost your well-being, one study found. Stopping to admire and snap a pic gives you a moment to be mindful. What's more, when the study participants looked for something different or unusual in their day, they seemed to have a greater sense of purpose, competence, and achievement. Plus, they exercised more.

Give it a shot (pun intended), and share an image every day for a week.

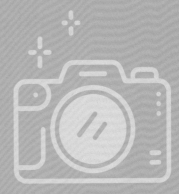

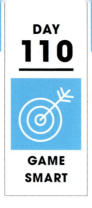

DAY 110 — GAME SMART

A haiku is a 3-line poem in which the first line has 5 syllables, the second line has 7 syllables, and the third line has 5 syllables. And yes, that's syllables, not words. Select an everyday object on your desk—a lamp, maybe, or your mouse pad—and **write an ode to it in the form of a haiku.**

DAY 111 **MENTAL HEALTH SMART**

Hug yourself. When you think negative thoughts about yourself, your brain's amygdala sends signals that increase blood pressure and raise adrenaline and cortisol levels. Try a "surreptitious self-hug" by wrapping your arms around yourself and squeezing. Even your own touch releases oxytocin and other feel-good biochemicals that promote well-being.

DAY 112 **BODY SMART**

Find your rhythm. Listening to music while you exercise makes a workout more fun and can add some bounce to your stride. So grab your smartphone and pop in some earbuds. If you're Spotify-savvy, create playlists of uptempo tunes to download onto your device.

Number Wheel

What number belongs in each empty space?

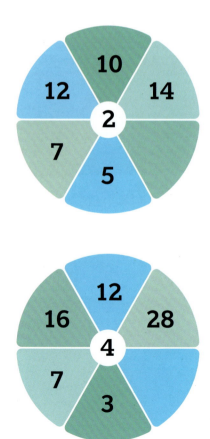

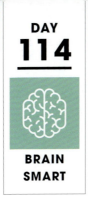

DAY 114

BRAIN SMART

Doing complex, intellectually challenging work may help keep dementia at bay. Think of 5 improvements you could make at work, either for your own position or for the company in general. Now take this idea to the next level: Try to execute at least one of those upgrades today.

Which improvements were you able to carry out at your workplace today?

_____

_____

_____

_____

_____

_____

_____

_____

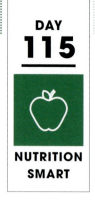

DAY 115 — NUTRITION SMART

Add in an egg or two today. Make an omelet for breakfast, a hard-boiled egg at lunch, or a frittata for dinner. Eggs deliver a double whammy of brain goodness. They're high in lutein and choline, 2 compounds that support brain development in children and overall cognitive function in adults. Choline is especially beneficial because it's needed to produce a neurotransmitter that plays an important role in memory, mood, and muscle control. And don't ditch the yolks! They not only taste great but are also where those nutrients live.

Fluffy salad and veggie topper
To add a hit of extra protein and some creaminess to your favorite cooked veggie or salad, grate some hard-boiled egg over the top just before serving.

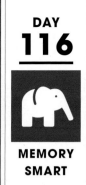

DAY 116

MEMORY SMART

IT'S YOUR CHOICE

Pick the memory strategy that works best for you. Try each strategy you've learned so far on these new lists. When you're done, commit to one strategy and make it a habit.

Resize It (Day 4) • **Rehearse It** (Day 11)
Label It (Day 32) • **Relate It** (Day 39) • **See It** (Day 53)
Tales (Day 60) • **Domino** (Day 82)

LIST A	LIST B	LIST C
3 7 4 9 7 0	RUT	TEST
U S 3 1 0 0 F	COVER	FABLE
5 T F 2 8 V W G	WEST	BOAT
	TABLE	POT
	TORN	FARM

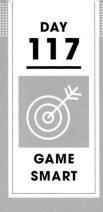

DAY 117

GAME SMART

Family Riddle

If Anna's daughter is my daughter's mother, **who am I to Anna?**

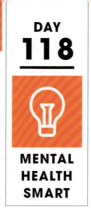

DAY 118

MENTAL HEALTH SMART

Here's an experiment to try: Banish all light from your bedroom tonight. The otherworldly glow from your phone isn't conducive to sleep, of course. But beyond that, even a little bit of light—like moonlight seeping through the slats of your blinds—can confuse your sleep system. Make the room as dark as possible. Will you sleep any better? If the answer is yes, try the next step: Think about investing in quality blackout shades, and buy an alarm clock with red or amber light, which will be less disturbing to your body's circadian rhythm than blue light.

What did you try? _____

_____

How did it work? _____

_____

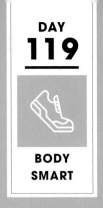

DAY 119

BODY SMART

Look for a drop-in beginner's yoga class nearby today.

Studies confirm clear benefits from yoga. In one, brain scans of women ages 60 and over who practiced yoga at least twice a week for an average of 15 years showed more activity in their prefrontal cortex (associated with attention and memory) than a control group of women who never did yoga. This suggests that yoga could protect against age-related cognitive decline, the researchers say. Another study indicates that 2 yoga sessions a week may **help ease symptoms of depression.**

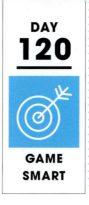

This game challenges your ability to identify similarities and differences within a group. Each of the symbols in the following set has 3 different characteristics in color, shape, and pattern. Find as many groups of 3 symbols as you can in which all 3 are either the same or different with respect to each of these characteristics.

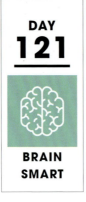

DAY 121 — BRAIN SMART

Try "batching" at work today. With this technique, you group similar tasks and then designate a specific time period to tackle them. Small administrative tasks could be scheduled for a time when you're low on energy, like midafternoon. For example, get all your emails done at once, all your calls, or all your invoices. Batching lets you focus on deeper work at other times—and you'll be more efficient and sharper overall.

What are 3 tasks you could batch?

_____

_____

_____

_____

_____

_____

DAY 122

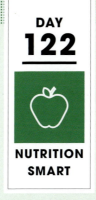

NUTRITION SMART

TODAY,

skip the alcohol. Make a spritzer by replacing some of the wine with sparkling water, and keep your alcohol consumption within the safe and healthful limit: **1 drink a day, max.**

The more alcohol a person drinks, the smaller his or her total brain volume becomes, one study found. And that link between drinking and reduced brain volume was stronger in women—probably because smaller people are more susceptible to alcohol's effects.

DAY 123

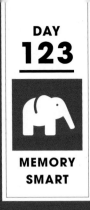

MEMORY SMART

Read the following list. When you finish reading, set your stopwatch for 2 minutes, cover the list with your hand, and write down as many items from the list as you can remember, in any order. Stop when the 2 minutes are up.

Pears	Cereal	Buns	Oranges
Cheese	Onions	Peas	Squash
Tuna	Pretzels	Bread	Ice cream
Beets	Waffles	Cabbage	Tape
Paper	Hot dogs	Yogurt	Plums

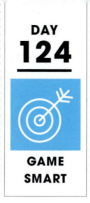

DIY Cube

Which of these cubes will the pattern shown create when folded?

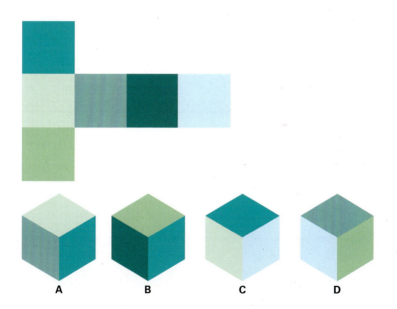

DAY 125

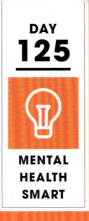

MENTAL HEALTH SMART

People who are conscientious— that is, self-disciplined and dependable—show less cognitive decline and fewer symptoms of Alzheimer's disease, research has found. That's good news, because you can cultivate conscientiousness. Nurture this trait: **Spend 20 minutes a day tidying up the house.**

DAY 126

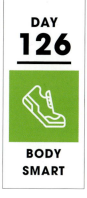

BODY SMART

Find a YouTube video and learn a new patterned dance—no partner required. Research suggests that learning and recalling a complex sequence of dance steps may not only challenge your leg muscles but also enhance your attention span. Dance styles requiring specific patterns of steps, such as ballroom or square dancing, offer your brain the most benefit.

Need some ideas? We'll get you started:

- Swing
- Waltz
- Foxtrot
- Tango
- Mambo
- Cha-cha
- Lindy hop
- Salsa
- Kizomba

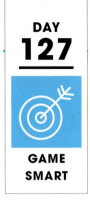

DAY 127 — GAME SMART

Color Confusion

Read aloud the colors of the words below—not what the words actually say! How long does it take? Can you do it faster a second time?

YELLOW   BLUE
WHITE   PURPLE
GREEN   WHITE
BLUE   GREEN
BLACK   GREEN
BLACK   RED
RED   YELLOW
YELLOW   BLACK

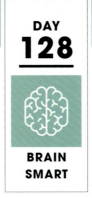

DAY 128

BRAIN SMART

This morning or evening, focus on the "far future," and think of the best possible outcomes for your social life, your life at home, and your career. First, grab a comfortable chair. Then, for 20 minutes, write in detail about these potentially happy outcomes—what your life would look like, what goals you would have met, and how you'd feel about yourself.

DAY 129

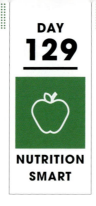

NUTRITION SMART

EATING PLENTY OF FISH AND SHELLFISH

can help keep your mind in top form and lower your risk of dementia, multiple studies suggest. Most scientists believe the benefit comes from the dose of omega-3 fatty acids you get with every bite of tuna or trout. Omega-3 fatty acids are powerful, versatile nutrients. Your body needs fatty acids of all different types from various foods.

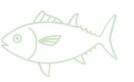

→ **This week, try these omega-3-rich fish:** Wild salmon, herring, tuna, sardines, Atlantic mackerel

DAY 130

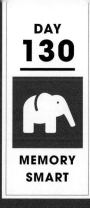

MEMORY SMART

Use the Rehearse It strategy from Day 11, and then the Resize It strategy from Day 4, to memorize these words. After you Rehearse It, close the book and write down as many words from the list as you can recall. How did you do? **Now try to remember the words using the Resize It strategy:**

Rock	Candle	Towel
Admire	Poster	Chime
Soap	Difficult	Log

DAY 131

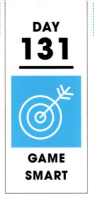

GAME SMART

Every day you use a brain skill known as deductive reasoning. That's the ability to reach a correct conclusion based on just a few existing facts. Here's an exercise that gives your powers of deductive reasoning a good stretch.

Can you read this message? Bet you can!

> GT N GRT SHP BY USNG TH BK.
> SRPRSE YRSLF AND YR FRNDS WTH
> YR PWRS OF DDCTV RSONNG. SM
> FMLIAR? PRHPS YOU OR YR KDS
> LK TO TXT MSSGE.

DAY 132

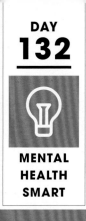

MENTAL HEALTH SMART

Tonight, crack a window while you sleep. It's no secret that a lumpy mattress or a snoring partner can lead to sleepless nights. But don't forget air quality: Poor ventilation can be an overlooked sleep stealer. Luckily, the solution might be as simple as opening a window or door, research suggests. To test whether a buildup of carbon dioxide as a result of respiration affected people's sleep, Dutch researchers tracked 17 volunteers over 5 nights. Some participants slept with a bedroom door or window open, while others did not. **The result:** The rooms with better ventilation had less CO_2 in the air, which seemed to translate to better slumber.

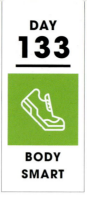

DAY 133

BODY SMART

Reward yourself for your workout today. When you complete your daily exercise, give yourself a new song download to add to your workout playlist. Or maybe buy a new workout shirt after your first month. You'll be surprised at how much an occasional self-pat on the back helps you to stay excited about that run, walk, or swim. **How will you reward yourself?**

_____
_____
_____
_____
_____
_____
_____
_____
_____

DAY 134

GAME SMART

Rebus Puzzles

What common phrase is each of these word pictures trying to say?

T_RN	~~SECRET~~
PLAY WORDS	SECRET SECRET

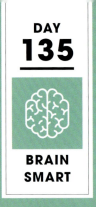

DAY 135

BRAIN SMART

Pick up a houseplant today.

Why? That little succulent sitting on your coworker's desk could be giving her a brain boost at work. In one study, employee productivity increased by 15% after plants were introduced to a previously bare office. In another, college students who performed demanding cognitive tasks in an office with greenery had longer attention spans than those in a plant-free office. **Our connection to plants may reduce stress and help us stay calm,** which in turn boosts our ability to be creative and focus on tasks.

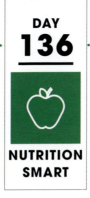

DAY 136 — NUTRITION SMART

Keep your blood sugar steady throughout the day by eating protein with each meal, and eating small, high-quality snacks. (Think whole-grain crackers, apples, and peanut butter.) You want to keep your brain's main source of fuel (glucose) steady. A blood sugar crash can make it a challenge to think clearly and get things done.

Today, note which protein sources took center stage in your meals:

_____
_____
_____
_____
_____
_____
_____

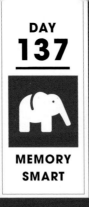

DAY 137

MEMORY SMART

Today, get a grip—for memory's sake. Clenching your fists may strengthen your memory now and improve your recall later, according to one study.

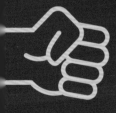

The technique: Clench your right fist the next time you're given a phone number to remember. Then clench your left fist when you're trying to recall that number. According to the study authors, the trick should work for different memory categories. Specifically, clenching your right hand appears to activate parts of your brain's left hemisphere, which is responsible for memory formation. Left clenching activates right-hemisphere regions, which are essential for recall.

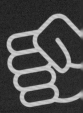

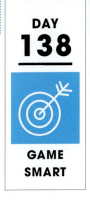

Cryptogram

For solving tips, see Day 190.

_ _ _
Y Q R

_ _ _ A _ _ _ S _
H C R I Y R X Y

_ _ A _ _ _
U R I G Y Q

_ S _
T X

_ A _ _ _ _
Q R I G Y Q

DAY 139

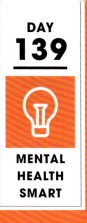

MENTAL HEALTH SMART

Worry wisely today. People who worry are really good at solving problems when those problems actually arise, according to research. The trick, though, is not to "pre-solve" every possible emergency, but only those you can deal with now. Some worry is productive—you want to finish presentation slides before a conference, or double-check your flight details—but most anxieties are about things that we can't control. If you can do something this minute to stave off a future event you're worried about, do it. If you can't, then give yourself a simple pep talk ("I'll be good at tackling that problem if it actually happens") and leave the worry behind.

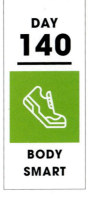

DAY 140

BODY SMART

Try a HIIT workout today. HIIT stands for high-intensity interval training, and its key principle is simple: 20 seconds of high intensity, followed by 10 seconds of recovery. After 4 minutes, take a full minute to rest. Repeat until you've been at it for 15 minutes. For some people, a power walk is their sprint. The key is to give it all you've got, and then walk in place for 10 seconds to recover.

What you do doesn't matter. You can jump rope, sprint up stairs, or do mountain climbers or squat jumps. In one study, HIIT participants lost weight and gained fitness and strength, of course. But they also had better short-term memory, longer attention spans, and clearer focus.

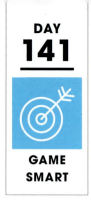

DAY 141

GAME SMART

This simple yet effective exercise trains your mental attention, speed, and flexibility. Connect the dots below in order, alternating between the 2 different sets of information (for example, A, I, B, II, C, and so on), working as quickly as you can. Be careful! Your mind needs to move back and forth between the 2 sets of information to complete the puzzle.

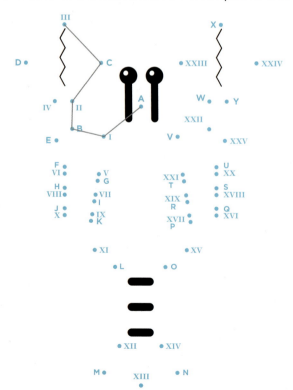

DAY 142

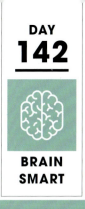

BRAIN SMART

Protect your noggin.

Although this book has offered many tips on saving your brain, you shouldn't overlook the obvious. If your feet aren't in contact with the ground—whether you're skiing, biking, rollerblading, or horseback riding—wear a brain-saving helmet. At home, move objects out of the way that might cause you to trip and fall. Stay off unsteady surfaces, such as ladders placed on uneven ground. **This last tip is obvious: Always buckle up in the car.**

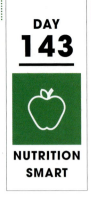

DAY 143 — NUTRITION SMART

Add some walnuts to your meal today. Mix them into a salad, sprinkle them on a dessert, or blend them up for a savory pesto. Chefs and nutritionists agree: It's crunch time. Walnuts have long been associated with better memory and brain function, especially when they're eaten as part of a Mediterranean-style diet. Where do the brain-boosting powers of walnuts come from? At least one study points to a specific group of antioxidants (polyphenolic compounds) that stomp out inflammation in brain cells. Here's an easy snack or appetizer that also packs a protein punch.

Apples with Honey-Yogurt Dip and Candied Walnuts

- **Combine** 1 tsp sugar and 1 Tbsp water in a small bowl.
- **Stir** to dissolve the sugar.
- **Place** 2 Tbsp walnuts in a small skillet and cook over medium-high heat, shaking the pan often, for 3 to 5 min., until lightly toasted.
- **Remove** the skillet from the heat and stir in the sugar mixture, tossing to coat.
- **Let cool.** Place ⅓ cup fat-free plain Greek yogurt in a small bowl and cover with 1 Tbsp honey and walnuts.
- **Serve** with 1 apple, sliced, for dipping.

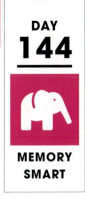

DAY 144 — MEMORY SMART

Stop trying to recall every grocery item or conversation and get in the habit of taking notes. **The Record It strategy** simply involves listing the items you need to recall. Take a few minutes to make a list of things you need in order to get something done. It could be a grocery list, to-do list, packing list, or checklist for a project at work.

DAY 145 GAME SMART

Find the Difference
Which number doesn't belong?

236   348   4416   5630   122

DAY 146 MENTAL HEALTH SMART

Commit to at least 10 minutes of self-care today. Even if it means locking the bedroom door and reading a chapter of an engrossing novel, you'll come away with a sense of control and accomplishment. What will you do for self-care today?

_____
_____
_____
_____
_____
_____

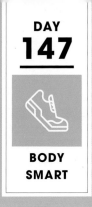

DAY 147

BODY SMART

Here's an exercise boost you can do at work, and it's really simple: If you have to communicate with anyone who sits within 500 feet of you, do it in person. Avoid the urge to call or email. Chances are they're feeling a little lonely at their desk around 4 p.m., too, so pop by and ask your question in person! They'll probably welcome the company, and you'll have an excuse to walk away from your desk. **Then write down who you visited with today:**

_____
_____
_____
_____
_____

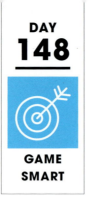

DAY 148

GAME SMART

Set your stopwatch for 3 minutes and solve as many of these math problems as you can. Feel free to use a separate sheet of paper for your calculations. Stop when the 3 minutes are up.

ROW

1. 7 x 4 =   21 + 32 =   149 - 45 =
2. 135 ÷ 5 =   40 x 8 =   3 x 8 =
3. 120 ÷ 10 = 24 + 5 =   70 - 7 =
4. 11 x 4 =   79 - 38 =   48 ÷ 2 =
5. 30 ÷ 2 =   53 - 11 =   32 - 7 =
6. 12 - 4 =   33 x 2 =   10 - 7 =
7. 4 + 17 =   27 x 5 =   85 ÷ 5 =
8. 92 - 5 =   66 ÷ 11 =   16 - 8 =
9. 101 - 40 = 209 + 12 =   81 ÷ 9 =
10. 54 + 21 = 40 - 3 =   43 + 29 =

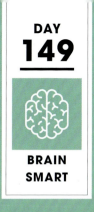

DAY 149

BRAIN SMART

Revisit your high school

or college language class. The ability to speak a second language may prime your brain to stay sharper as you age. Individuals who've spent several years speaking 2 languages on a daily basis are speedier when switching between tasks than their monolingual peers are, research reveals.

Being proficient in a second language over a long span of time appears to be key for a sharper mind.

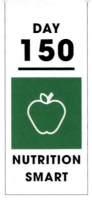

DAY 150

NUTRITION SMART

EAT YOUR VITAMIN E

with breakfast, lunch, or dinner. You'll find this vitamin in such foods as nuts and seeds, vegetable oils, and fortified breakfast cereals. **High levels of vitamin E are associated with improved cognitive performance** and have been found to reduce the risk of Alzheimer's-related functional decline.

DAY 151

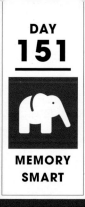

MEMORY SMART

REMINDER FILE: Keep better track of all those dates and times you need to remember. Get a large manila envelope and label it "Reminder File." Put the envelope in a convenient place, such as on your desk or the table where you sort mail. As things arise that you need to remember (a lecture at the library, concert tickets you need to order), write yourself a note and put it in your Reminder File. Once a week, go through the Reminder File and log all your entries into your appointment book. Stick with this plan, and you'll never miss another event.

Where will you store your reminder file?

_____

Which day of the week will you go through it?

_____

DAY 152 **GAME SMART**

Number Pattern
Which number is missing from this series?

11 13 17 ___ 23 29

DAY 153 **MENTAL HEALTH SMART**

Meditate for 15 minutes today on your lunch break or before you leave for work. Sit up straight, close your eyes, and focus on what you're experiencing in the present moment, whether it's birds chirping in the distance or just the sound of your own breathing. In one study, scientists noted cerebral cortex growth among meditators. (The cerebral cortex is an area of the brain that controls memory, language, and sensory processing.) In another, meditators performed better than their non-meditating counterparts on a series of mental acuity tests.

When will you meditate today? _____

DAY 154

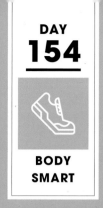

BODY SMART

Exercise boost!

Today, speed it up while you exercise. One study found that exercisers who did two 3-minute sprints memorized new words 20% faster afterward than those who skipped the workout. Research shows that cardio exercise increases blood flow, triggering growth in the area of the hippocampus responsible for memory and verbal learning.

If you walk or jog on a treadmill, amp up the speed. If you walk or jog outdoors, note how long it takes you to complete a section of your usual route—say, 4 laps around the block. Now quicken your pace and try to do 5 laps in the same amount of time.

DAY 155 — GAME SMART

Solve the following trivia question:
Before Mount Everest was discovered, what was the highest mountain in the world?

Answer: _____

DAY 156 — BRAIN SMART

Listening to music increases concentration and productivity in office workers and improves attention and cognition in people with dementia. Stop what you're doing and cue up a favorite song. Listening to a song you love lowers levels of the stress hormone cortisol, which can otherwise impede cognition.

DAY 157

NUTRITION SMART

At lunch, get your fork out for an arugula salad.

Arugula is a nutritional standout among greens: It's very high in nitrates, which are compounds that increase blood flow to the brain by dilating blood vessels. A serving size is roughly 2 cups raw—about the size of a salad. In one study, people who ate a serving or two of leafy greens a day had the cognitive abilities of someone 11 years younger than people who ate none. If your brain isn't getting enough blood flow, it's also not getting enough oxygen, which can result in cell death.

DAY 158

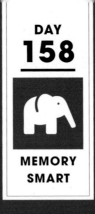

MEMORY SMART

Remember those memory tricks you learned a few weeks ago? Read the lists below and see if you can apply your favorite technique. When you finish reading, **set your stopwatch for 2 minutes** and write down as many listed items as you can remember, in any order. **Stop when the 2 minutes are up.**

LIST A	LIST B	LIST C
3 7 4 9 7 0	RUT	TEST
U S 3 1 0 0 F	COVER	FABLE
5 T F 2 8 V W G	WEST	BOAT
	TABLE	POT
	TORN	FARM

DAY 159 — GAME SMART

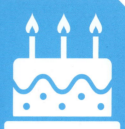

Number Riddle
Linda is 54 years old and her mother is 80. How many years ago was Linda's mother three times her age?

DAY 160 — MENTAL HEALTH SMART

Tonight, try a natural sleep inducer by jumping in the tub. Taking a bath before bed relaxes your muscles and releases muscular tension—and it has a chemical effect as well. While you're in the tub, your core body temperature will rise. Then when you get out, it will quickly drop. **Why is that good?** The temperature dip signals your brain to release melatonin.

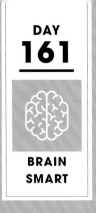

DAY 161
BRAIN SMART

HERE'S A CHALLENGE:

Toss a ball while you walk. Why is the brain a booster? In a study from Germany, adolescents who bounced, threw, or passed balls with alternating hands for just 10 minutes showed better attention and concentration in a subsequent lesson and test. You don't have to be a kid to enjoy this benefit, the researchers say. **Their theory is that handling a ball primes the part of your brain that controls focus.**

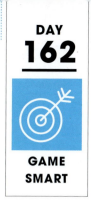

DAY 162

GAME SMART

See how many triangles you can find in the drawing below.

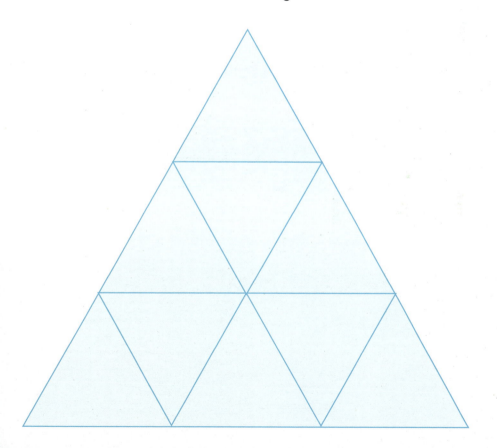

DAY 163

BRAIN SMART

Plan a trip. Almost nothing challenges your brain like navigating a new locale, and research links travel to stronger cognitive health. If you can't hop on a flight to a far-off land, be a tourist in your own city by strolling through a new-to-you neighborhood or spending the afternoon at a large museum. In general, novel experiences will always engage your brain in healthy ways.

Brainstorm some possible destinations—near and far—below:

_____
_____
_____
_____
_____
_____
_____
_____

DAY 164 **NUTRITION SMART**

Drink peppermint tea. A common remedy for nausea, peppermint tea has also been found to improve long-term and working memory in healthy adults. Researchers found that peppermint tea drastically enhanced long-term memory, working memory, and alertness, compared with hot water and chamomile tea (which actually slowed memory and attention speed).

DAY 165 **MEMORY SMART**

Test yourself. On your way to the grocery store or any other store you might need to visit today, try to recall your entire shopping list. This is a test of your working memory, or your ability to keep and recall information in the presence of distractions. Even though it won't make you smarter, working memory comes in handy every day—like keeping a grocery list in mind as you comb the shelves.

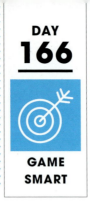

Mystery Word Search

Find the names of six healthy foods in the grid below.

V	B	F	S	O	N	P	R	X	I
C	A	E	L	A	K	H	B	G	S
W	N	R	Y	A	L	I	R	N	Z
L	A	S	E	T	D	K	O	O	P
H	N	L	O	W	J	A	C	M	E
B	A	C	N	M	G	S	C	L	Q
E	P	U	Q	U	I	N	O	A	U
N	K	E	C	R	T	L	L	S	O
T	I	A	R	G	Y	H	I	W	K
S	T	N	A	F	D	D	S	U	E

DAY 167

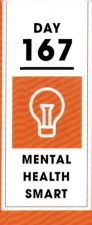

MENTAL HEALTH SMART

Help out at an animal shelter or walk a neighbor's dog. Multiple studies show that time spent with dogs or cats can bolster your emotional and even physical health. To get some of that love (even if you can't have a dog or cat), you could volunteer at an animal shelter or sign up with a dog-walking service. And even if it's a critter you're just getting to know, the payoffs are similar to those you'd get from having your own pet. Spending time with furry friends both old and new carry some of the same health benefits, such as potentially lowered blood pressure.

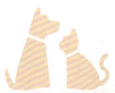

DAY 168

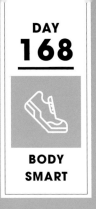

BODY SMART

BRUSH YOUR TEETH 3 TIMES TODAY,

after breakfast, lunch, and dinner. Oral health is clearly linked to brain health, according to a team of British psychiatrists and dentists. After studying thousands of people between the ages of 20 and 59, they found that gingivitis and periodontal disease were associated with worse cognitive function throughout adult life—not just in later years.

DAY 169

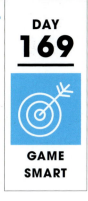

GAME SMART

Math Logic

Using the information in the first 3 grids, what is the missing number in the final grid?

2		1
	24	
3		4

4		3
	96	
4		2

8		3
	48	
1		2

5		2
	?	
2		4

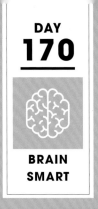

DAY 170

BRAIN SMART

Today,

place your phone out of sight if you need to get something done. Your brain's ability to hold and process data is compromised whenever a smartphone is within reach, even if it's powered off.

In fact, a 4-second interruption—the time it takes to glance at your phone—can triple your chances of making a mistake during a task.

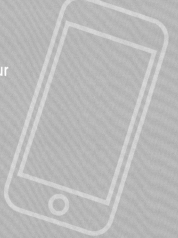

DAY 171

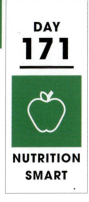

NUTRITION SMART

Pack your plate with cruciferous vegetables. This family includes broccoli, cauliflower, cabbage, kale, bok choy, and brussels sprouts. These plants with emerald-green foliage are chock-full of antioxidants such as vitamin C, along with pigments called carotenoids. Some research suggests that eating steamed broccoli, a spinach salad, or other cruciferous vegetables or greens may actually help turn back the clock on your "brain age." One 25-year study showed that women who ate the most leafy greens and cruciferous vegetables lowered their brain age by 1 to 2 years.

What did you eat today?

_____
_____
_____
_____
_____

DAY 172

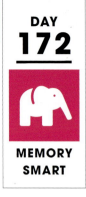

MEMORY SMART

Establish a Memory Place. Find a bowl, dish, or other container that's large enough to hold your keys, wallet, glasses, phone—any important object that you're constantly picking up and putting down (and can't find later). Set up your Memory Place near your front or back door—whichever entry you use most often. Now cultivate the positive habit of always putting those frequently lost objects in your Memory Place. Here's another useful idea: Keep a pad of sticky notes and a pen in your Memory Place. That way, when you remember something you need to take with you (like the dry cleaning or a book to return), you can write yourself a note and stick it on the door.

Where will your memory place be, either in your home or at work?

_____

_____

_____

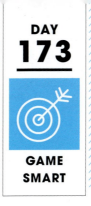

DAY 173 — GAME SMART

Visual Math

What number does each fruit represent?

🍏 + 🍏 + 🍓 = 70

🍏 + 🍓 + 🍓 = 50

🍏 + 🍓 + 🍊 = 60

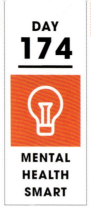

DAY 174

MENTAL HEALTH SMART

FRAME A PHOTO OF A HUG.

Images of people being supported or loved can dial down your brain's threat response, research suggests. When study participants were shown huggy photos, alarming words and images of unfriendly facial expressions no longer made the amygdala (the brain's threat monitor) light up. Researchers say that displays of social support tap into this brain response—even when they take place between strangers in a picture.

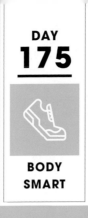

DAY 175

BODY SMART

Today, try a walking meeting. Leave the conference room behind, and you just might get more done. Not only do walking meetings get your energy up, but stepping outside with your coworkers creates a sense of equality that may help resolve problems better. **After all, nobody's at the head of the table.**

DAY 176

GAME SMART

Hone your brain's visual flexibility by learning to look at the same object from different perspectives. Can you picture this? And that? Each of these 3 pictures depicts 2 very different images, depending on how you look at it. Can you see both?

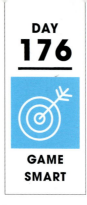
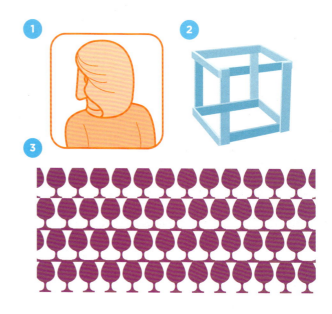

What are they?

1. _____
2. _____
3. _____

DAY 177

BRAIN SMART

Schedule your tough upcoming task between 11 a.m. and 2 p.m. That's when levels of the sleep hormone melatonin dip sharply from their late evening and early morning peaks, meaning you're more ready to take on projects, say researchers in Germany. Last year, they found that reaction time and the ability to accomplish several to-dos were strongest in the middle of the day. So tackle your errand list, voicemails, or emails. Give a presentation to a client or boss, or iron out a tough problem with your spouse. Because of your mental quickness, this time of day is best for getting things done.

What could you get done today?

_____

_____

_____

DAY 178

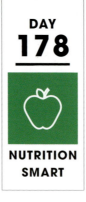

NUTRITION SMART

Cut down on foods not included in the MIND diet, which emphasizes antioxidant-rich berries, vegetables (especially leafy greens), whole grains, and fish. (The omega-3 fatty acids in fish are thought to help your brain's nerve cells communicate with one another). Try to reduce your intake of foods that contain saturated and trans fats, both of which may damage your cardiovascular system and, by extension, your brain health. That means less red meat, butter, margarine, pastries and other sweets, and fried or fast foods. Older people who stuck with this style of eating over 5 years were able to lower their Alzheimer's risk by 35% to 53%, research found. The longer people stayed on the diet, the more their odds improved.

Below, write down a list of your favorite MIND foods and circle 2 you'll eat today.

_____

_____

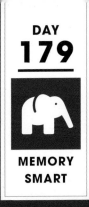

DAY 179 — MEMORY SMART

Make a habit of the Morning Minute.

Every morning, take 1 minute to look at your calendar and to-do list. This simple step forces you to review and pay more attention to your appointments and errands. **Most important, it makes you more likely to remember them once your day starts cooking.**

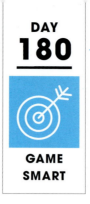

DAY 180 — GAME SMART

That's a Wrap

List as many alternate uses for a newspaper as you can think of, such as swatting flies, packing fragile items, or making papier-mâché crafts.

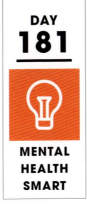

DAY 181

MENTAL HEALTH SMART

Today, plan a quick outing with a friend or family member, or perhaps someone you'd just like to know better. People who spend lots of quality time with family members, friends, and other social contacts are more likely than reclusive people to retain a keen wit and healthy brain as the years pass. In fact, research reveals that memories of social butterflies can be twice as strong as those of people who spend little time with friends and loved ones. The scientists also estimate that Alzheimer's risk can be double among people who say they often feel lonely. **Who could you hang out with today?**

_____
_____
_____
_____

DAY 182

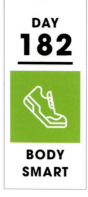

BODY SMART

Here's a good way to break up the day and sneak in a workout. First, head to a nearby set of steps. Now try a pushup on the second or third step: Hands shoulder-width apart, toes on the floor at the bottom of the stairs, feet hip-width apart. Slowly lower your chest by bending your elbows 90 degrees. Descend as far as you can, and then slowly rise back to your starting position. If you're a beginner, you can do a modified version by starting with your knees on the floor.

The regular way
Do 2 sets of 12 pushups.

Make it easier
Do 2 sets of 12 modified pushups.

Make it harder
Do 3 sets of 12 pushups

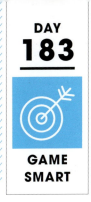

DAY 183

GAME SMART

Fill in the blanks with the numbers or letters that come next in the sequences.

ROW									
1	3	7	11	15	19				
2	2	9	16	23	30				
3	A	D	G	J	M				
4	1	A	3	C	5	E			
5	ff	i	tt	f	ii	t			

DAY 184

BRAIN SMART

Time crunch!

If you do the daily crossword in your local newspaper, give yourself the goal of completing it in under 30 minutes. If that becomes too easy, cut your time to 25 minutes.

Or

play another timed smartphone game. The best way to boost your brain skills is to play against a clock. The pressure of time ticking away shifts your attention, processing speed, and other brain skills into overdrive. The faster they need to work, the more your brain skills will improve.

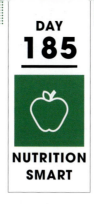

DAY 185

NUTRITION SMART

Caffeine isn't the only part of a cup of java that makes you sharper. There's magic in the beans themselves, even decaf beans. Coffee beans contain compounds called phenylindanes, which studies suggest may give your brain health a lift by preventing the buildup of proteins believed to contribute to the development of dementia and Alzheimer's.

Coffee Slushie: In a blender, puree 8 oz coffee, 1 Tbsp chocolate-hazelnut spread, and 1 cup ice until smooth.

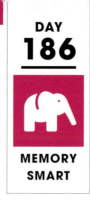

DAY 186 — MEMORY SMART

Today, learn how to prep for memory stress. If you're about to speak publicly, have a talk with your boss, or otherwise deal with an intense moment, know that stress hormones, such as cortisol, may chemically block your ability to recall some information—just when you need it most. To handle a stressful event that requires memory, use these strategies to stop cortisol confusion:

- **Sip a cup of tea or java.** Animal studies suggest that moderate amounts of caffeine may enhance long-term memory when taken shortly after learning.
- **Do a last-minute review.** Researchers think that memories are not affected by cortisone (cortisone is used by the body in the production of cortisol) on same-day tests. It's likely that the "freshness" of the memory can overcome the stress.
- **Take a deep breath (or two).**
- **Try to relax.** A short stroll, a friendly conversation, or deep breathing before the big event may help keep stress hormones in check.

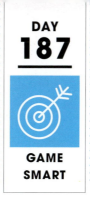

DAY 187

GAME SMART

Word Finder

Connect adjacent letters to find the superfoods listed below. One letter can connect to the next in any direction, and a letter can be used for more than one word. Bonus: Write out the remaining letters to discover a related word.

E	H	F	E	A
K	L	I	S	L
T	A	H	H	X
E	B	N	A	I
E	S	F	L	R

- KALE
- BEANS
- FISH
- FLAX

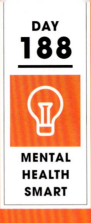

DAY 188

MENTAL HEALTH SMART

Today, try an exercise one physician prescribes to all her patients, which she calls "5 by 5": Set an alarm to go off at 5 intervals throughout the day, and dedicate 5 minutes to stopping all brain activity. Don't even meditate! Just be in the moment. You might close your eyes and take a rest, or sit outside and look at trees. Go for a walk (without listening to a podcast!) and zone out. **Just 5 minutes with no major input is the best way to reset your brain.**

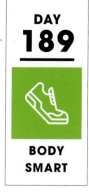

DAY 189

BODY SMART

GET UP FROM YOUR DESK EVERY 40 MINUTES TODAY.

Your office provides plenty of excuses. Print to the farthest printer from your desk, investigate whether the bathrooms on the floor above you really are nicer, do a quick sun salute before your morning meeting. You get the picture. If you're so in the zone that hours go by and you're still glued to your chair, set an alarm on your computer. If that's not a productive way to fill your calendar, we don't know what is.

Tally how many times you got up and moved around today?

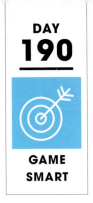

Cryptogram

In a cryptogram, or secret code puzzle, each letter in the original message is replaced by another letter in a specific pattern. (For example, the word YES can be encrypted to XDR by replacing each letter with the one before it: Y with X, E with D, and S with R.)

To start, figure out which words are logical in the grammatical structure of a sentence (THE, ON, OF, and so on).

Solving this puzzle will reveal a famous quote composed of 11 words, plus the author's name.

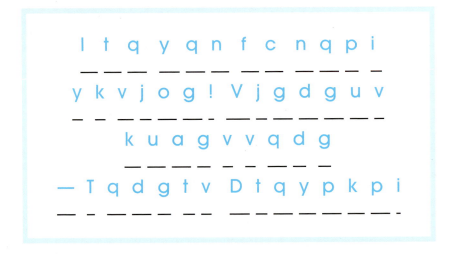

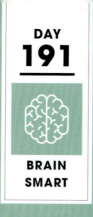

DAY 191
BRAIN SMART

Do a kind thing for a family member today to increase positivity, and don't bicker or criticize.

Older adults who had negative social support—that is, relatives or friends they considered unreliable, critical, or aggravating—were up to 31% more likely to develop dementia, according to British researchers who followed more than 10,000 people over age 50 for more than a decade. Those who had positive support from spouses or children were 17% less likely to show signs of mental decline over the years.

What's something kind you can do for a family member, or a compliment you can give?

_____

_____

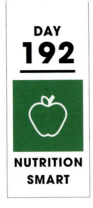

DAY 192

NUTRITION SMART

Head to the store or farmers' market and put blueberries in your basket. Bring 'em home to sprinkle over your cereal or yogurt or fold into your smoothie. Off-season, go with frozen berries, which are every bit as nutritious as fresh. These purple nuggets may help sharpen your thought processes. In one study, rats that ate blueberries showed increased cell growth in the hippocampus region of their little brains. The researchers believe that anthocyanin—the dark blue pigment in blueberries—is behind those cognitive changes. Anthocyanin contains chemicals that may cross the blood-brain barrier and lodge in regions that govern learning and memory, they explain. **Get your daily dose with the smoothie recipe below,** which includes 1 cup of blueberries, along with other proven brain health boosters. (Spinach, anyone?)

Love-Your-Brain Smoothie: Blend 1 cup **blueberries**, ¾ cup **water**, ½ cup **spinach**, ½ cup **yogurt**, ¼ cup **coconut milk**, 1 tsp **matcha powder**, and ½ tsp **turmeric**, adding **ice** as needed, until smooth.

DAY 193

MEMORY SMART

Take an inventory of your junk drawer for a visual memory workout. Open the drawer and study the contents for 1 minute. Then close the drawer and write down as many items as you can recall.

Want a brain-boosting bonus? Reorganize the drawer and toss out the genuine junk.

DAY 194

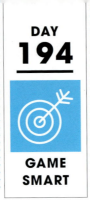

GAME SMART

Coded Message

Use the coordinates here to fill in the quote from William James.

A: a1, a4, b2, c2, c6

C: a2, d7

D: b7, c7, e4

E: c4, d3, d5, d8, e6

F: a7, d1, d2

H: b1

I: a6, c8, e2

K: c3

M: c1

N: d6

O: b5, b8, e5

R: d4

S: a5, c5, e7

T: a3, b3, e3

U: b6

W: a8

Y: b4

.: e1, e8

	1	2	3	4	5	6	7	8
a								
b								
c								
d								
e								

DAY 195

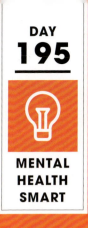

MENTAL HEALTH SMART

Are you a slumberjack, sawing logs? Pick up the phone and book an appointment with your health care provider, who may send you to a sleep specialist. Raise-the-rafters snoring is no mere annoyance—especially if the racket is punctuated with gasps, snorts, or long pauses between breaths. These are symptoms of sleep apnea, a condition of disrupted breathing and sleep that studies have linked to an increased risk of brain disease. If you're diagnosed with sleep apnea, you'll likely end up with a prescription for a continuous positive airway pressure (CPAP) machine. **This is an effective therapy that can restore normal breathing.**

DAY 196

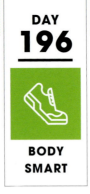

BODY SMART

Here's a good way to break up the day and sneak in a 5-minute workout, and all you need is a set of steps. Stand on the floor facing the steps. Leading with your left foot, step up on the first step while driving your right knee up (as if you're trying to hit your chest). Return both feet to the floor. Do this 12 times, and then switch feet (lead foot to the right, drive up with the left knee).

The regular way
Do 2 sets of 12 step-ups with each leg.

Make it easier
Do 1 set of 12 step-ups.

Make it harder
Do 3 sets of 12 step-ups.

DAY 197

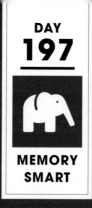

MEMORY SMART

Set your stopwatch for 2 minutes and write down as many words that begin with B as you can. Do not repeat words and avoid using proper names. Stop when the 2 minutes are up.

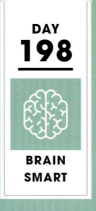

DAY 198

BRAIN SMART

Today,

close your eyes when doing a safe everyday task (as in brushing your teeth, not chopping onions!). Your brain relies on a combination of sensory information from your limbs, joints, and eyes to coordinate movements.

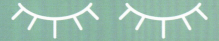

By closing your eyes, you force your brain to adapt. This improves something called plasticity, which is your mind's ability to make adjustments when faced with new experiences. That process tends to wane with age.

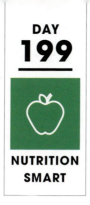

DAY 199

NUTRITION SMART

Today, say no to sugar to get a better night's sleep and a brainier day tomorrow.

Postmenopausal women who consumed lots of refined carbs (especially added sugars) were more likely to develop insomnia, according to researchers who analyzed food diaries.

Those who ate more fiber-filled produce were less likely to toss and turn at night. Why? Refined carbohydrates, such as sugar, white flour and rice, can spike blood sugar, prompting the release of insulin to lower it. **Once your blood sugar levels dip, stress hormones like adrenaline and cortisol flow, which may mess with your sleep.**

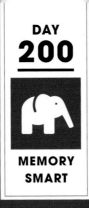

DAY 200 — MEMORY SMART

Do you remember the skills you learned earlier? Let's find out. Describe in a few words these memory strategies:

Resize It

Rehearse It

Label It

Tales

Videos

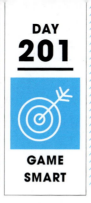

DAY 201 — GAME SMART

Shape Sudoku

Using the six shapes below, fill in the grid so that no shape is repeated across, down, or within the marked rectangles.

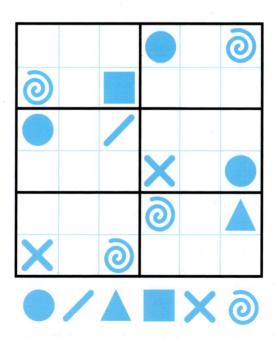

DAY 202

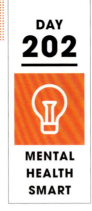

MENTAL HEALTH SMART

Can't concentrate? When you worry about something today, think of one small thing you can do to address your worry, even if it's just talking to a friend, and do it. Taking small, positive actions reduces the mental stress that destroys concentration and bathes your brain in harmful stress hormones. Taking action can also stimulate healthier brain function.

What's something you're worried about today?

_____

_____

_____

What's something you can do to address the worry?

_____

_____

_____

DAY 203 — BODY SMART

Feeling like your workout has been too easy lately? Getting a bit bored? Try ramping up the intensity. If you work out on a treadmill, raise the incline. If you walk or jog outdoors, add some hills or stadium steps to your route.

DAY 204 — GAME SMART

Do the Math

How can you use one **1** and four **7s** to create the number **100**? You can use any mathematical operations (such as +, −, ×, ÷).

DAY
205

BRAIN SMART

Today, tap into creative solutions between 9 a.m. and 11 a.m. This is the time when your brain has moderate levels of the stress hormone cortisol, which in reasonable amounts can help your mind focus. It's present at any age: One study found that both college students and retired adults were mentally quick in the morning—although among the older participants, sharpness declined in the afternoon.

**Take on tasks that require analysis and concentration.
Here are some ideas:**

- Develop a new idea.
- Write a presentation.
- Brainstorm solutions to address challenges large or small.
- Have an important conversation with your doctor.

What are some tasks you could do today?

_____
_____
_____
_____

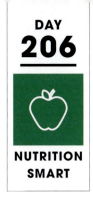

DAY 206

NUTRITION SMART

Back on Day 10, we encouraged you to drink more water to keep your brain in play. How's that going? If you're getting bored with basic water, try these creative infusions:

Cinnamon Water
This spice isn't just for cookies. Drop a cinnamon stick in your glass for a dose of its blood-sugar-stabilizing benefits, and you just might beat that afternoon slump.

Melon Water
Pick your favorite melon, grab your spiralizer, and crank out some ribbons of fruit for a pretty and refreshing pick-me-up. Bonus: At 90% water, melon can rehydrate you and restore your fuel reserve of glycogen after a workout.

Orange-Rosemary Water
Mix in some orange slices and a sprig of rosemary to add a nice touch of earthy flavor to your usual citrus sipper. Better yet, research suggests that rosemary can enhance memory and help you stay alert.

Blackberry-Sage Water
Give your brain a boost with this delicious drink. Blackberries pack antioxidants that prevent inflammation and help with motor skills. And sage is a known memory booster.

DAY 207

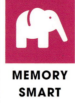

MEMORY SMART

Add a study period today. Remember back in school when you'd study 5 hours the night before a test, but remember next to nothing a week later? Try spending an hour each night studying any material, like next week's presentation or a wedding toast. You'll not only be prepared for your big moment but are also likely to remember that info years later.

Is there anything you could study tonight that will give you an edge on next week?

_____

_____

_____

_____

_____

DAY 208

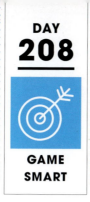

GAME SMART

Missing Letters

What single 3-letter sequence will complete all these words?

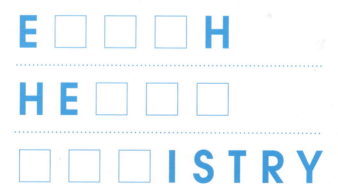

E ☐ ☐ ☐ H

HE ☐ ☐ ☐

☐ ☐ ☐ ISTRY

DAY
209

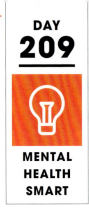

MENTAL HEALTH SMART

Today, look up volunteer opportunities. When you lend a hand for a cause you believe in, that sense of purpose and connection could bring big benefits. Whether you read to preschoolers, cook at a local soup kitchen, or help rake an older neighbor's yard, you could get a sneaky bonus: better health and happiness.

In one study, people who gave 100 hours or more a year were 28% less likely to die from any cause than their less altruistic peers. And a 5-year study found that recent retirees who volunteered for at least an hour a week on a regular basis were nearly 2½ times less likely to develop dementia than those who didn't volunteer.

If you don't have a go-to activity, head to volunteermatch.org for ideas. You could be a film festival docent or even assist a woman who's preparing to give birth. (It's searchable by location, interest, or age group.) You can also ask about volunteer opportunities at your local school, place of worship, or Red Cross chapter. Then write down your ideas and research below:

___

___

___

DAY 210 **BRAIN SMART**

Improve your sequencing skills by answering this question:

How many times does the number 4 appear in the numerals 1 to 100?

DAY 211 **GAME SMART**

Here's another opportunity to stretch your mind with a new and unusual challenge. Write a mystery novel—in 10 words or less.

_____
_____
_____
_____
_____
_____

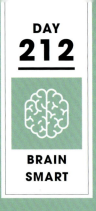

DAY 212 — BRAIN SMART

Nix the noise

in the workplace (or at home), by wearing earplugs today. Ringing phones and noisy copiers are problematic enough, but the real potential harm comes from the conversations you can barely overhear. It's not clear exactly why this is, but one theory is that your brain automatically wants to channel its mental resources toward understanding speech. That means less brainpower devoted to your own thoughts.

> **You can probably pick up a good, soft pair of earplugs at the drugstore for around a dollar.** Or plunk down the cash for a set of active noise-canceling earbuds.

DAY 213

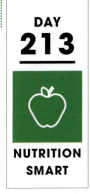

NUTRITION SMART

Snacking on celery and green bell peppers may help keep your mind sharp. Luteolin, a plant compound abundant in these green vegetables, can help prevent brain inflammation that's linked not only with aging but also such diseases as Alzheimer's and multiple sclerosis, researchers say. The scientists studied the compound's effect on human brain cells in a test tube and on mice; in both cases, it decreased inflammation.

Try dipping celery and green bell pepper slices in hummus, or make a healthy tuna salad: Mix chopped celery and peppers, herbs (like parsley and chives), tuna, and a dollop of plain yogurt.

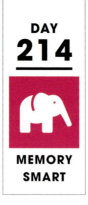

DAY 214 — MEMORY SMART

Improve your reading skills today. Ever feel like you're missing the point of a story, or have a hard time remembering the story? Try this approach, called Straight Story:

1. Pause. Stop for a few seconds and focus your thoughts.

2. Identify the main point. All stories are hierarchical: That means some information in a narrative is more important than other information, and that at some point in the tale you'll discover the essential ingredient. How can you find it? Figure out the phrase or plot point that's so critical that the rest of the narrative makes no sense without it.

For example, in the movie *Titanic*, the main point is that the ship hit an iceberg and sank. Think about it: If the ship stays afloat, the romantic intrigue and the other subplots don't really matter.

3. Don't let minor details sidetrack you. Let your mantra be "Just the facts, ma'am—and only the really important ones." You'll remember the details anyway, once you've got the main point down.

4. When you've identified the main point, go back and add a few of the major details to get to the heart of the story.

Using *Titanic* again, you would add to the main point (the ship sank) by focusing on the lost lives. You still wouldn't focus on the romantic intrigue—but I bet you'd remember that detail anyway.

5. Try the Straight Story technique with stories you read today in the newspaper or online.

DAY 215

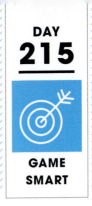

GAME SMART

Word Fill-In

What's the longest word you can come up with that starts with the letter on the left and ends with the letter on the right?

B _____ G

R _____ A

A _____ M

I _____ E

N _____ S

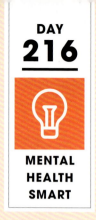

DAY 216

MENTAL HEALTH SMART

Visit an aquarium,

whether you go in person or virtually. Focusing on marine creatures—in a tank, at an aquarium, or even on a livestream—can soothe anxiety. In a 2016 study at the U.K.'s National Marine Aquarium, people's heart rates slowed within 5 minutes of watching a tank filled with water. As fish were added, they slowed even more.

In another study, participants showed a significant reduction in cortisol levels and blood pressure after walking through an immersive, naturalistic exhibit. Ever consider getting a tank at home? You might get some of that same fish-watching relief.

DAY 217 **BODY SMART**

Here's a counterintuitive move: End your workout at a slower pace. Concluding your run with a slow jog, for example, may help you get moving again tomorrow. In one study, people who ended their workout at a pace that was slower than their starting pace thought their sessions were more pleasant than people who raised the intensity as they went along (even though both groups did the same amount of work). More important, they didn't dread their next get-moving session and even thought it would make them feel good.

DAY 218 **GAME SMART**

Reading + Math
If you tore out pages 24, 25, 26, 41, 42, and 67 from a magazine, how many sheets of paper would you be holding?

DAY 219

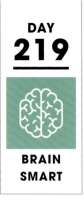

BRAIN SMART

Visit your local toy store and check out the different brands of handheld electronic games, such as Hasbro's Simon, which provides a great cross-training brain workout at a low cost. Get into the habit of playing whichever game you choose several times a week for at least 10 minutes. Before you buy, make sure a product challenges your attention span, speed, and flexibility—and becomes more challenging as your skills improve.

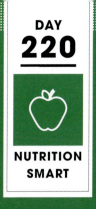

DAY 220

NUTRITION SMART

Today, choose organic.

Eat a variety of fruits and vegetables to reduce your exposure to any one particular pesticide, and shop organic whenever possible. Always wash produce under running water. Before you wash lettuce or other leafy vegetables grown with pesticides, toss the outer layer, where residue accumulates.

DAY 221 MEMORY SMART

Call a friend you haven't spoken to in at least 3 years. Or contact an old classmate through Facebook. As you reminisce, you'll probably end up talking about mutual friends you knew in the old days. That's a great booster for your memory bank.

DAY 222 GAME SMART

Missing Piece
Which shape will fit in the space?

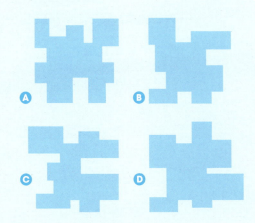
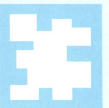

DAY 223

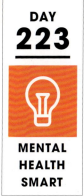

MENTAL HEALTH SMART

Do one thing that makes you happy and optimistic about the future—your outlook may affect your Alzheimer's risk. In a U.K. study, older adults answered questions about negative thinking patterns, depression, and anxiety, and also had cognitive function assessments and brain scans over 2 years. People with higher levels of repetitive negative thinking patterns, such as ruminating about the past and worrying about the future, showed more cognitive decline and memory problems. They were also more likely to have brain deposits of amyloid and tau, which are proteins linked to Alzheimer's. Repetitive negative thoughts are linked to factors believed to contribute to these deposits.

What's one thing you can do today to help you look forward to the future?

DAY 224 — BODY SMART

Take your blood pressure at a local pharmacy or supermarket, if you haven't done so in a while. Physical activity increases blood and oxygen flow in the brain, while high blood pressure can damage small blood vessels there. To lower your Alzheimer's risk, exercise regularly and maintain a normal blood pressure.

DAY 225 — BRAIN SMART

If you work at home, create a schedule to improve your focus. While more of us have learned to work from home, that doesn't mean we're doing it in the healthiest or most productive way. Shut down your work computer by 7 p.m. every night, and set a morning schedule. For a big productivity boost, change out of those pajamas first thing in the morning, and get into some can-do clothes.

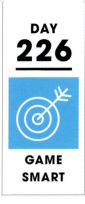

DAY 226

GAME SMART

Set your stopwatch for 1 minute and study the photograph below. When the time is up, turn to the next page. Write down as many objects as you can remember from the photo you just studied.

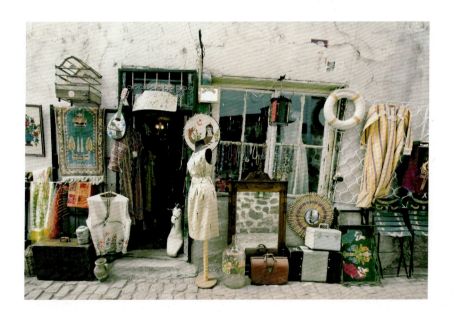

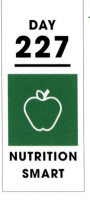

DAY 227 — NUTRITION SMART

EAT SOME PROBIOTIC-RICH YOGURT TODAY.

Researchers believe that gut microbes may directly affect neurotransmitters, sending signals from your stomach to your mind. In one small study, women who ate probiotic yogurt had decreased activity in the area of the brain that controls emotion, cognition, and sensory feelings in response to an emotion-recognition test. Those who consumed no probiotics had an increase in activity, meaning they reacted more to the negative images. Yogurt is a protein-rich snack with a big nutritional payoff, so dig in. Your brain might just reap a benefit too. **Other fermented products,** such as wine, some naturally brewed beers, and cheese, are also sources of probiotics.

DAY 228

MEMORY SMART

Get into the habit of taking notes whenever you receive critical information. Taking notes is especially important when you're meeting with a doctor, lawyer, or financial planner, or in any other weighty circumstances. Stress and anxiety can cloud your memory. Note-taking is always a good idea on the job, too.

Try this: Staple several sheets of blank paper to the inside of a project folder and use them to take notes during meetings or client calls. Later on, you can go back to these notes for a record of what you discussed.

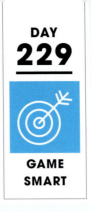

DAY
229

GAME SMART

Mystery Word Search

Can you find 3 grains, 3 greens, and 3 fruits?
Words may be vertical, horizontal, or diagonal.

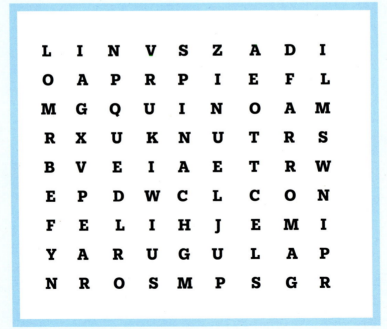

DAY 230 **MENTAL HEALTH SMART**

Give your brain a massage. Relieving tension via acupressure points may help regulate the hypothalamus, the part of your brain that controls hunger and stress hormones. To curb food cravings, use both hands to massage both sides of your spine where your hairline meets your neck. Do it for 2 to 3 minutes.

DAY 231 **BODY SMART**

If your oven is on, open a window or door every half hour and turn on the ventilation fan above your stove. Gas stoves and appliances can produce carbon dioxide. While researchers have long believed that carbon dioxide is relatively harmless, one small study suggests that carbon dioxide can mess with your brain's ability to reason and make decisions.

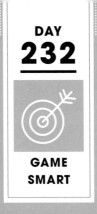

DAY 232

GAME SMART

Today you will try a

deceptively simple task

that requires attention, ingenuity, creativity, and—perhaps above all—a steady hand. Grab a deck of playing cards and use them to build a house. (You might want to close the window first! A breeze could wreck it all.) Not as easy as it looks, is it?

DAY 233

BRAIN SMART

Today, try journaling. Writing is one of the best brain-stimulating activities because it forces you to assimilate information: You have to plan what you'll say, organize it, write it down, and edit it. This requires attention, concentration, and sequencing, all of which strengthen your brain, especially your memory. In one study, people who completed three 20-minute scribe sessions over 2 weeks showed significant improvements in their working memory. **Try waking up 15 minutes early to document your thoughts and feelings while your mind is still fresh.**

_____
_____
_____
_____
_____
_____

DAY 234

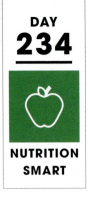

NUTRITION SMART

Today, swap low-quality carbs for high-quality carbs. The first things to limit are sweets and soda, of course. Highly processed carbohydrates (such as white bread, white rice, bagels, and some cold breakfast cereals) quickly convert to sugar. Get your fizzy drinks by flavoring sparkling water with a splash of fruit juice, and eat more "good" carbs. These include quinoa, whole grains, yams and other vegetables, beans, and fruit, to name a few. They raise your blood glucose levels more gradually.

Which carbs did you swap out today?

Low Quality

_____
_____
_____
_____
_____

High Quality

_____
_____
_____
_____
_____

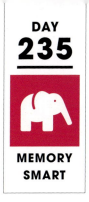

DAY 235

MEMORY SMART

Always forget

where you parked? Today, try this 2-minute memory trick. Believe it or not, breathing through your left nostril may help, say researchers in India. Adults ages 20 to 45 who practiced this yoga technique had a 16% boost in spatial memory, which is key for navigating complex parking lots or garages. Experts believe there's a link between the nostril you breathe through and parts of the brain that control memory.

Try this

Gently press your right thumb against your right nostril. Inhale and exhale through your left nostril 27 times. **Repeat up to 4 times a day.**

DAY 236

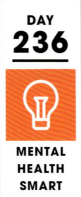

MENTAL HEALTH SMART

Do you ever feel like the noise in your head interferes with your focus and concentration?

Learning to be mindful of the details in the world around you is a great way to strengthen your ability to sustain attention. (It's an effective stress buster too.) Take a 5-minute stroll in a familiar place. But instead of letting your thoughts drift to worries and daily concerns, focus on what's going on around you. At the end of your walk, write down five things you saw that you'd never noticed before.

1. _____
2. _____
3. _____
4. _____
5. _____

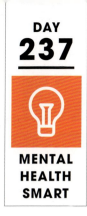

DAY 237

MENTAL HEALTH SMART

Work near a window.

That's because if your desk is close to daylight, you may sleep better at night. Workers with windowed spaces slept about 46 minutes longer each night than those who were not exposed to natural light in the workplace, one study found. Light has a big influence on maintaining an in-sync circadian rhythm. Chronic circadian disruption can make you feel run-down, crabby, hungry, distracted, and sad, and it may even play a part in heart disease, cancer, obesity, and depression.

DAY 238 — BODY SMART

Having a hard time listening lately? Schedule a hearing exam—or at the very least, turn that racket down. If you're one of the 31 million Americans with hearing problems, your memory may be suffering, too. Research shows that people with hearing loss sometimes spend so much effort trying to understand what's being said that they can't remember it afterward. Have your hearing tested every 3 years after age 50. Prevent further hearing loss by turning down the volume on your devices.

DAY 239 — GAME SMART

Rebus Rally
Each of the word combinations below represents a common phrase. Can you figure out all three?

1. eggs
   easy

2. sell
   buy

3. scotch
   rocks

DAY 240

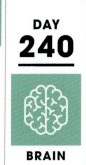

BRAIN SMART

Look for a brain-building class. Have you ever thought about taking a literature course at your local college and finally learning the nuances of Faulkner and Fitzgerald? If fiction's not your thing, maybe you're a history buff or a budding botanist. Or perhaps it's opera, ornithology, or origami that intrigues you. A number of studies have linked learning and brain health: The more years you spend immersed in academic pursuits, the longer you're likely to remain sharp, lucid, and free of cognitive disease. Scientists theorize that the mental stimulation of getting an education allows some people to build stronger brains and blunt the symptoms of dementia.

Look into local university continuing education programs, community colleges, and the Osher Lifelong Learning Institute (If you're 50 or older). Thanks to the internet, many classes are now offered online or via Zoom, too. **Write down some options today:**

_____

_____

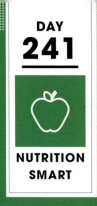

DAY 241 — NUTRITION SMART

Eat your B12 today.

Getting adequate amounts of this B vitamin, found in animal products and fortified foods, helps reduce levels of homocysteine, an amino acid linked to cognitive impairment. In a study of older adults with elevated homocysteine levels and memory problems, B vitamin supplementation improved memory and reduced brain atrophy.

Which of the following foods can you eat today?

- ☐ Sockeye salmon
- ☐ Nutritional yeast
- ☐ Clams
- ☐ Beef liver
- ☐ Milk
- ☐ Rainbow trout
- ☐ Cereal (fortified with B12)
- ☐ Tuna
- ☐ Octopus
- ☐ Crab

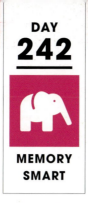

DAY 242
MEMORY SMART

Today, intentionally allow your mind to wander after taking in new information. Giving your brain a little time to space out after absorbing new information can help improve storage and recall, research finds. When your brain is not working on a specific task, it uses its idle time to sort and store memories.

So letting your mind wander—even for a few seconds—after reading an interesting article or attending a lecture could help you better remember the details later on.

DAY 243

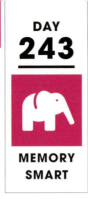

MEMORY SMART

Name Recall

List the middle names of everyone you'll see at Thanksgiving this year. (Don't know them? Conversation starter!)

_____

_____

_____

_____

_____

_____

_____

_____

_____

_____

_____

_____

DAY 244 MENTAL HEALTH SMART

If worries, fears, or nagging what-ifs are intruding on your mental health, show them the exit. As soon as you recognize an intrusive negative thought, visualize a stop sign. You can even say "Stop!" aloud, if it helps. Or wear a rubber band around your wrist to "snap" yourself out of it.

DAY 245 BODY SMART

If a set of stairs is nearby, practice some triceps dips. Here's how: Sit on the edge of a step with your hands at your sides and feet flat on the floor. Push your butt off a step, bend your elbows, and slowly lower your body toward the floor. Keep your butt close to the step, brushing it on the way down. Return to the starting position.

The regular way: Do 2 sets of 12 dips.
Make it easier: Do 1 set of 12 dips.
Make it harder: Do 3 sets of 12 dips.

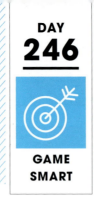

DAY 246 — GAME SMART

Using one set of information in different ways tests your brain's flexibility. How many words can you make out of each of the words below?

Balderdash

Cacophony

Onomatopoeia

DAY 247 **BRAIN SMART**

Switch your ringer off if you need more focus. Research shows that "song" ringtones are the most disruptive to productivity, followed by a more standard ringing sound. No song, less distraction.

Bonus move: Send out an office memo to see if everyone will agree to set their cellphones to vibrate during the day. You'll probably get more thanks than grumbles from your coworkers.

DAY 248 **NUTRITION SMART**

Enjoy a square of dark chocolate today. Dark chocolate has been shown to boost blood flow to the brain, and as little as a third of an ounce a day may help protect against age-related memory loss. Bonus: Chocolate also stimulates the release of certain feel-good chemicals in your brain called neurotransmitters. So you'll not only plow through those emails like a boss, but you also just might do it with a smile.

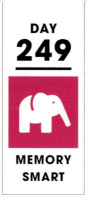

DAY 249 — MEMORY SMART

Try using the Straight Story technique from Day 214 with a TV show or movie you watched in the past week. Write down your answers below.

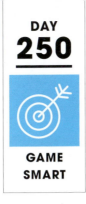

DAY 250 — GAME SMART

Study this painting for a few minutes. What details do you notice? Close the book, do something else for a while, and then return and study the painting again. **Are there any details you didn't notice the first time?**

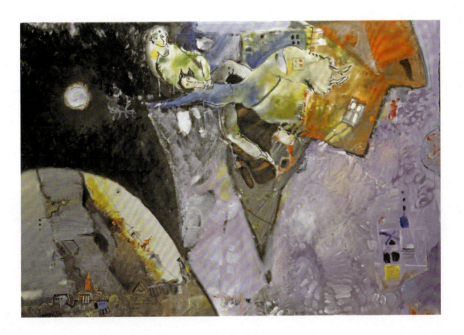

DAY 251 **MENTAL HEALTH SMART**

Enjoy some morning light today. Early-morning light suppresses production of the sleep-promoting hormone melatonin and syncs your body clock with the time of day. The result? You're more alert. Every region of your brain and body has its own inner clock. Bonus points: Get your light while on a morning walk.

DAY 252 **BODY SMART**

If you've been feeling forgetful, review your medications with your health care provider. Many prescription drugs can affect your memory, and the older you are, the longer drugs stay in your system. Medications that can affect memory include antidepressants, anti-anxiety drugs, beta blockers, chemotherapy drugs, Parkinson's drugs, sleeping pills, painkillers, antihistamines, and statins.

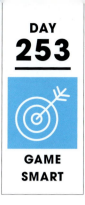

DAY
253

GAME SMART

Add to the Top

If each circle contains the sum of the two numbers below it, what is the top number? (Challenge: Can you do it in your head without filling in the circles?)

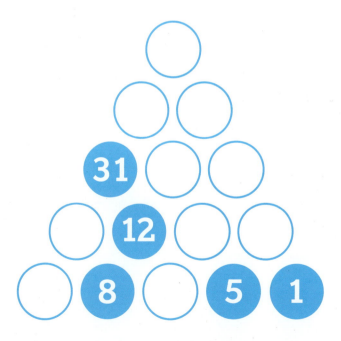

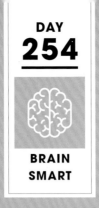

DAY 254

BRAIN SMART

Declutter for clarity today.

Research shows that clutter can make it harder to concentrate. By contrast, when finding things is a breeze and you're not overwhelmed by disorganized mess, you're less anxious. After the piles of yesteryear's shoes and kitchen gadgets have been put away or donated, try rearranging your furniture or giving your home a mini-facelift. That may give you a renewed sense of control over your surroundings.

DAY 255 **NUTRITION SMART**

Today, drink a cup of tea, whether it's hot or cold. A recent study associated a high intake of flavonoid-rich foods and beverages, such as tea (19 cups a month) with a lower risk of Alzheimer's and dementia. Flavonoids, which are found in abundance in tea—especially green tea—likely play a role, thanks to their anti-inflammatory properties.

DAY 256 **MEMORY SMART**

Use one of the memory techniques from this book to learn some new names or phone numbers. Write down information you'd like to learn here (your doctor's phone number, your mother-in-law's birthday, your work email password, or that nice neighbor's name). Then practice.

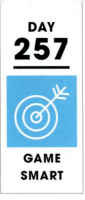

DAY 257 — GAME SMART

Odd One Out
Which one of these gloves doesn't have a match?

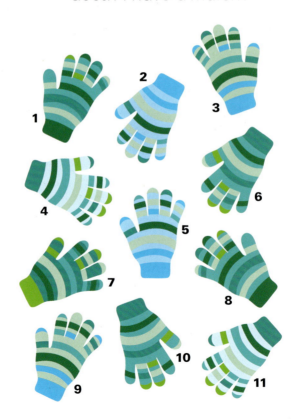

DAY 258

MENTAL HEALTH SMART

Invite someone over for dinner tonight.

Brain health is compromised by social isolation, and stress may fuel inflammation that wreaks havoc on memory. Having someone over for pasta or stir-fry fosters conversation and a sense of closeness, both of which relieve inflammation-inducing stress.

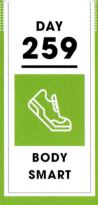

DAY 259

BODY SMART

Think you're not a morning person?

Use these tips today to prep for a morning workout tomorrow:

- **Plan to exercise with a friend.** You'll be less likely to hit the snooze button if it means standing someone up.

- **Lay out your gym attire.** Some people even sleep in their workout clothes!

- **Place your alarm clock across the room,** so you're forced to get out of bed to turn it off.

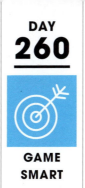

Missing Math

Which math symbols could you add between these numbers to make each equation correct?

a) 1 2 3 4 = **4**
b) 4 3 2 1 = **3**
c) 4 3 2 1 = **2**
d) 1 2 3 4 = **1**

DAY 261

BRAIN SMART

Today, do a Google search or ask friends on Facebook to find a nearby book club. A little peer pressure to finish a book by a certain date can go a long way, especially if you're expected to talk about the content. Budget the number of pages you'll need to read each day, and if you own the book, write notes in the margin and mark meaningful passages to boost your concentration and comprehension.

DAY 262 **NUTRITION SMART**

Just say no to sugar all day today and see if your memory improves. If you can't remember where you put your keys, that cookie might be to blame. According to a recent study, elevated blood sugar levels are damaging to both long- and short-term memory.

DAY 263 **MEMORY SMART**

Try using the **Straight Story** technique from Day 214 again, with a play or musical you've seen on stage. Write down your answers below.

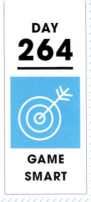

Missing Piece

Which puzzle piece will fit in the empty spot?

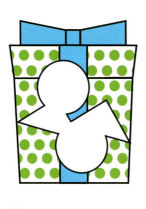

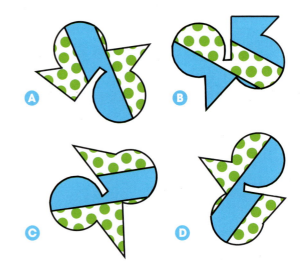

DAY 265

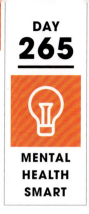

MENTAL HEALTH SMART

Snooze this afternoon. Quality restful sleep is non-negotiable when it comes to thinking fast on your feet. As you progress from slow-wave sleep in the first part of the night to REM sleep in the early morning hours, your memories transform the material you learned throughout the day into actual working knowledge. There's no substitute for getting those 7 to 8 hours. But a strategically timed nap can come surprisingly close.

When you nap in the middle of the day, your time in each stage is more efficient. In a 90-minute nap, you cycle through both slow-wave and REM sleep, but you do it in the same proportion as it occurs across a whole night of sleep. Because of this, a 90-minute nap can rival what you'd get overnight in terms of memory consolidation, creativity, and productivity. Too hard to fit 90 minutes into your schedule? A 30-minute nap can help lock in information, too.

When could you sneak in a catnap?

_____

_____

_____

_____

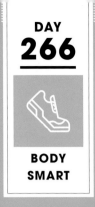

DAY 266

BODY SMART

Ten-hut!

Find a boot camp class today. Agility drills, like those in a tough but fun boot camp class, challenge and train both body and mind, research confirms.

All exercise can stimulate neuron development, but people who did agility exercises for 6 weeks—think high knees, mini-hurdles, cone drills, and fast feet—had greater increases in memory and alertness than those who stuck with calisthenics and running.

If boot camp isn't your thing, there's always Zumba, step aerobics, or yoga. Workouts that push you to pay attention and completely concentrate on balance and coordination will deliver more of a memory boost than monotonous activity.

DAY 267

GAME SMART

Spot the Symbol

Hone your visual searching skills with this table featuring many different symbols. Count how many times the three symbols at the top appear in the entire table, spending 30 seconds on each.

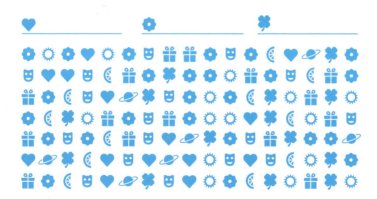

DAY 268

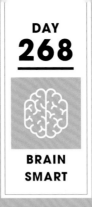

BRAIN SMART

Make sure you're reading for results today.

Ever found yourself rereading a page or spacing out mid-text? To reverse this habit, try these tips:

- **Read actively.** Take time-outs to process the material; mentally recap plot points or a character's motive, for example.
- **Read backward for a bit.** If you glossed over a few paragraphs, read them in reverse. That helps, because reordering small packets of information can sometimes change how much of it you absorb. It may feel odd at first, but the extra effort required will force your brain back into focusing.
- **Give up on dull books!** As you might expect, studies show that you're most likely to drift when you're not interested in the material. If a book doesn't grab you after a chapter or two, choose a new one.

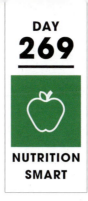

DAY 269 — NUTRITION SMART

Today, try to eat lunch closer to 2 p.m.,

as the midday meal can make you wish there were a couch close by. To digest your lunch, your body draws blood away from your brain and to your stomach.

Your body's circadian rhythm (the biological clock that regulates your sleep and wakefulness) is also in a brief "down phase" during this time. Use the time to meditate, pray, read a magazine, check the news, or visit websites. If you're at work and need to fight off drowsiness, go for a quick walk around the block or drink some water—both will get your blood moving away from your stomach and toward your head.

DAY 270

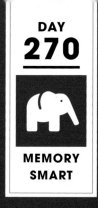

MEMORY SMART

Here's another **memory hack** to try today. Expert memorizers use a technique called Memory Palace, where they mentally store a word in a different area of their house.

To recall the list, they simply visualize themselves taking a stroll through their house. It's a tip used by servers at high-end restaurants, who don't want to scribble down people's orders on a pad of paper.
You can also use it to remember a grocery list.

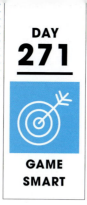

DAY 271

GAME SMART

Write down as many types of animals as you can think of in 1 minute. How did you do?

_____
_____
_____
_____
_____
_____

Now try this exercise again, only this time pick your own category—car models or flowers, perhaps.

_____
_____
_____
_____
_____
_____

DAY
272

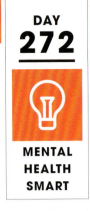

MENTAL HEALTH SMART

Redirect your attention toward the good things you're doing for your well-being. Maybe you've stuck with your walking routine, or replaced cookies with fruit for dessert. Thank your body for what it can do. More focus on the good stuff will help you feel more upbeat and satisfied in general and can even improve your sleep. **Can you list the things you've done for yourself lately?**

_____
_____
_____
_____
_____
_____
_____
_____
_____

DAY 273 **BODY SMART**

Try stationary cycling. A small but promising study found that people who logged 30 minutes on a stationary bike had better ability to recall names than others who simply rested.

DAY 274 **GAME SMART**

What's Missing
Which of the circles below belongs in this sequence?

  ?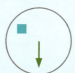

    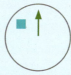

A   B   C   D   E

251

DAY 275

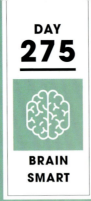

BRAIN SMART

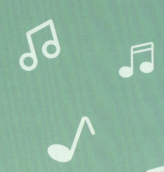

LOOK FOR MUSIC LESSONS NEAR YOU.

Taking up an instrument as an adult may feel daunting, but it's definitely doable, experts say. Research shows that making music can reduce your stress, lower your blood pressure, and decrease your heart rate. It also has a surprising effect on reaction time: While most people tend to have slower reactions as they get older, people who play an instrument react more quickly to both sound and touch.

The idea is that training the senses to work together can strengthen the sensory neural pathways and create brain-level benefits. If playing music for long periods of time improves reaction times by significant amounts, it's possible that learning to play an instrument in middle age or later could also have similar but less pronounced benefits.

Recreational music schools or community colleges typically offer adult beginner classes, or you can search in your area for a private teacher for one-on-one instruction.

DAY 276 **NUTRITION SMART**

Still battling sugar cravings? Today, instead of eating that pint of ice cream, try one of these fixes:

- Whole-wheat toast (check for no added sugar) + cream cheese + berries
- Freeze-dried banana chips + cacao nibs
- Almonds + dried goji berries + toasted coconut flakes
- Sweet bell pepper slices + guacamole

DAY 277 **MEMORY SMART**

Today, try "n-back," a Concentration-like memory game using cards. Here's how to do it: Lay a pair of face cards (king, queen, or jack) facedown. Now, flip two over as you look for matches. As you improve, try to play with the face cards as well as the numbers 7 and above. Then do all cards from 2 to ace. You can work your way up to play with the whole deck as you look for all four aces, kings, and so on.

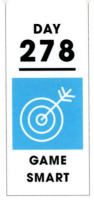

DAY 278 — GAME SMART

Missing Number Square

What two-digit number belongs in the empty square?

12	16	26
50	52	32
43	?	77

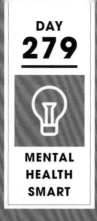

DAY 279

MENTAL HEALTH SMART

Find a new wake-up tune for a perkier start to your day. The sound of your alarm could affect the way your day begins, one study suggests. After the researchers had people fill out a detailed questionnaire about sleep inertia—also known as morning grogginess, which can affect daytime performance—they found a connection between waking to harsh alarm tones, such as beeping, to increased morning grogginess. Melodic tunes, on the other hand, seemed to improve alertness.

Abrupt sounds, the scientists speculate, may disrupt or confuse brain activity during waking, making you feel less than refreshed. More research is needed to determine what an ideal alarm sounds like, but for now, it can't hurt to set yours to something sweeter.

DAY 280

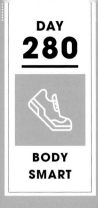

BODY SMART

Shake up your exercise routine!

If you've been using 5-pound weights for most strength exercises and usually finish the last rep with ease, it's time to go heavier. For your next workout, increase the weight of your dumbbells by 2 or 3 pounds. If you've been stopping at 8 or 10 reps, consider doing 12 reps on the easier moves.

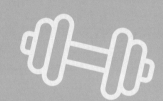
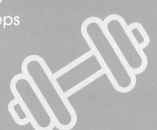

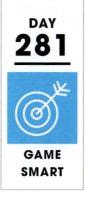

Building Blocks

Which is the only correct square?

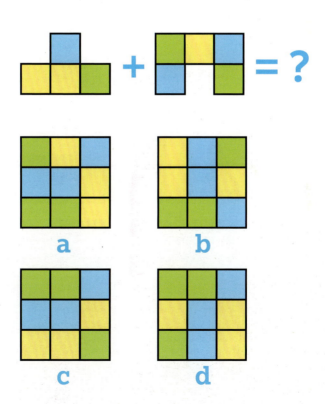

DAY 282 **BRAIN SMART**

Tonight, take apart a TV show. Dissecting the information you encounter in top-down, effortful ways can keep your memory sharp, research indicates. So after the show is over, try to distill what you just saw into parts. What was the point of the episode? What growth did the characters experience? How would you rewrite the ending? If you give your brain work to do, you'll keep your memory sharp.

DAY 283 **NUTRITION SMART**

Pop some raspberries (fresh or frozen) into your yogurt, cereal, or smoothie today. Berries are bursting with antioxidant compounds called anthocyanins, which have a unique ability to cross the blood-brain barrier. Simply put, those raspberries have good stuff that actually enters your brain, grabs free radicals, and escorts them out.

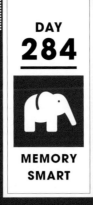

DAY 284

MEMORY SMART

Today, review your memory tools

and organization strategies. At a minimum, you should be using a scheduler, such as a Google calendar or appointment book, and a to-do list. **Which of these memory tools do you use?**

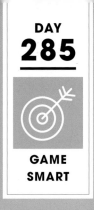

DAY 285

GAME SMART

Cryptogram
In this cryptogram, or secret-code puzzle, each letter in the original quote is replaced by a numeral in a specific pattern. (For example, the numbers 1, 2, and 3 could be encrypted to A, B, and C by replacing each number with the letter that corresponds to its order in the alphabet.) Exercise your deduction skills by solving this one to reveal a well-known quotation from Shakespeare.

"21·16   3·6,   16·19   15·16·21   21·16
__ __   __ __,   __ __   __ __ __   __ __

3·6:   21·9·2·21   10·20   21·9·6
__ __: __ __ __ __   __ __   __ __ __

18·22·6·20·21·10·16·15."
__ __ __ __ __ __ __ __."

For solving tips, see Day 190.

DAY
286

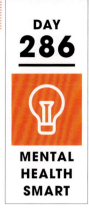

MENTAL HEALTH SMART

If Day 62's tip hasn't inspired you to start a gratitude journal, consider this a chance to check in with what you're thankful for. Write down 3 to 5 things you're grateful for today. Research indicates that building gratitude may bolster resilience by reducing feelings of hopelessness and powerlessness. Remember: **Be specific.**

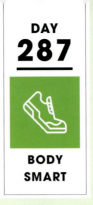

DAY 287

BODY SMART

Find out where you can learn tai chi.

This type of martial art is marked by slow, gentle movements and deep breathing, and it provides the perks of movement along with stress reduction and mindfulness. The results can be powerful: Research shows that tai chi is just as good as talk therapy (and better than medication) at helping breast cancer survivors deal with insomnia.

If your local YMCA or community college doesn't offer a class that works with your schedule, check out the Tai Chi for Health Institute (taichiforhealthinstitute.org) to find workshops or classes near you.

Practicing with a group will provide more motivation than going it alone at home, but there are also great video options to choose from, including *Anthology of T'ai Chi & QiGong: The Prescription for The Future*.

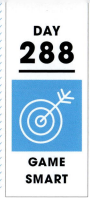

DAY
288

GAME SMART

Multiply This

Can you replace the remaining numbers from 1 through 9 in the empty spots so that the problem is correct?

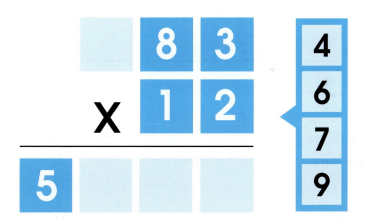

DAY 289

BRAIN SMART

Do some self-teaching online today. When you go googling, you engage key centers in your brain that control decision-making and complex reasoning. Spend about 20 minutes searching topics you've always wanted to know more about. Don't worry about how frivolous the topic seems: Whether you're looking for a celebrity's latest pratfalls or tips on musical harmony, the benefits to your brain are the same. **Write down a few topics you want to research today.**

_____

_____

_____

_____

_____

_____

_____

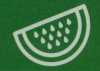

DAY 290

NUTRITION SMART

Refuel your electrolytes. Electrolytes are minerals that have an electric charge. Once they're in your body, they do double duty:

They balance the amount of water in your body to help your cells function properly, and they spark nerve impulses. Electrolytes also help you stay hydrated. When you sweat, you lose sodium, potassium, calcium, magnesium, phosphate, and chloride along with water. Without enough of these minerals in your body, you're not able to retain the water you're chugging during workouts or on a hot day; this could lead to dehydration. Being well hydrated keeps your electrolytes where they need to be, and certain snacks help, too. Bananas, spinach, milk, and yogurt are all good sources of electrolyte minerals. A sweet potato sprinkled with sea salt is another good option.

More electrolyte-charged foods: watermelon, avocado, almonds, oranges, and beets

DAY
291

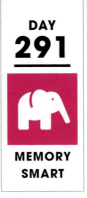

MEMORY SMART

Test Your Memory
Can you remember your last 7 meals?

DAY 292

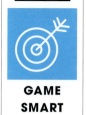

GAME SMART

Set your stopwatch for 3 minutes and solve as many of the following math problems as you can. Feel free to use a separate sheet of paper for your calculations. Stop when the 3 minutes are up.

ROW

1. 7 x 4 =   21 + 32 =   149 - 45 =
2. 135 ÷ 5 =   40 x 8 =   3 x 8 =
3. 120 ÷ 10 = 24 + 5 =   70 - 7 =
4. 11 x 4 =   79 - 38 =   48 ÷ 2 =
5. 30 ÷ 2 =   53 - 11 =   32 - 7 =
6. 12 - 4 =   33 x 2 =   10 - 7 =
7. 4 + 17 =   27 x 5 =   85 ÷ 5 =
8. 92 - 5 =   66 ÷ 11 =   16 - 8 =
9. 101 - 40 = 209 + 12 =   81 ÷ 9 =
10. 54 + 21 = 40 - 3 =   43 + 29 =

DAY 293

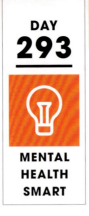

MENTAL HEALTH SMART

How happy are you at work? Write a list of things to explore in your career, big or tiny: One might be "Update LinkedIn"; another, "Explore the growing medical technician field." Your list does not have to be perfect. You're just opening your mind to possibilities.

Then make a move. Do at least one list item each day and build up to more. Some may seem silly and you might have to step back to move forward. (For example, you can't jump into that new tech field without going back to school first.) But that's okay: Resilient people are flexible with goals.

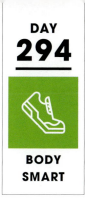

DAY 294 — BODY SMART

Get in some extra steps at lunch.

Get out today! Running to the deli downstairs means you'll get back to your desk faster, but a few extra minutes of walking could make a big difference. Try that new Thai place a few blocks away, or take your lunch to a park within walking distance and eat in the sunlight instead of under dreary fluorescents.

Where will you go (or where did you go) at lunch?

_____
_____
_____
_____

Bird's-Eye View

Which image below is the view of this pyramid from above?

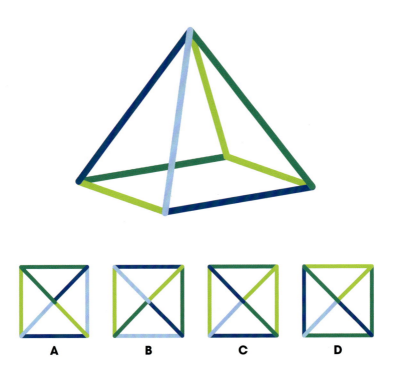

DAY 296 — BRAIN SMART

Shake up your environment to give your brain a fresh challenge. Has it been years since you reorganized your desk or closet? Get out of that rut and rearrange your work space. Now you'll have to think before you reach for the stapler or sweater.

DAY 297 — NUTRITION SMART

Try turmeric in one meal today. This spice is rich in curcumin, a potent anti-inflammatory. In a small study, people without dementia who took 90 mg of it twice a day showed better memory and attention compared with those who took a placebo. Try to cook with turmeric twice a week. You'll find turmeric in many Indian dishes, and turmeric lattes in many cafes.

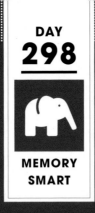

DAY 298 — MEMORY SMART

Today, practice learning a new name.

One of the most effective ways to remember names is to adopt the Rehearse It strategy you learned on Day 11: That is, repeat a person's name as soon as you hear it. Not just once, but don't repeat it so often that you seem weird. For instance, if you're at a party and a woman tells you her name, you might say, "Eliza? Hello, Eliza, it's a pleasure to meet you." Then introduce Eliza to someone else for another mention!

DAY 299

GAME SMART

Line Drawing

Can you trace over this image without ever lifting your pencil or going over the same line twice?

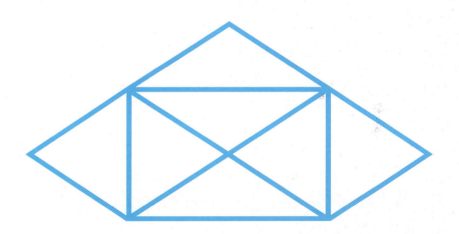

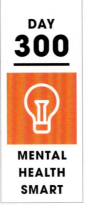

DAY 300

MENTAL HEALTH SMART

Fall asleep

to "pink noise" tonight. Researchers have found that this relaxing kind of background sound—rain falling or leaves rustling, for example—can help boost memory during deep sleep. In a study, pulses of pink noise were delivered to participants over age 60 during the stage of sleep when the brain stores the day's learning in long-term memory. Upon waking, the people who had been exposed to pink noise performed better on memory tests than those who hadn't been exposed.

Good news:

Most sound machines (and apps) offer both white and pink noise.

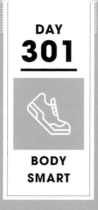

DAY 301

BODY SMART

Call your provider today

for a cholesterol check. A healthy cholesterol level is as essential for mental sharpness as it is for cardiovascular efficiency. When plaque, caused by LDL (bad) cholesterol, builds up in blood vessels, it can hinder circulation to your brain, depriving it of essential nutrients. One possible consequence is memory problems. Also, several studies point to high cholesterol as a risk factor for Alzheimer's disease. While that connection is not fully understood, the take-home is clear: Get your cholesterol checked regularly. If it's high, work with your doctor to lower it.

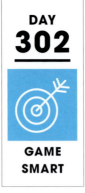

DAY 302

GAME SMART

Order by Number

Read the clues below and figure out the three-digit number.

682
One digit is correct
and in the right spot.

614
One digit is correct
but in the wrong spot.

153
No digits are correct.

296
Two digits are correct
but not in the right spot.

839
One digit is correct
but in the wrong spot.

___ ___ ___

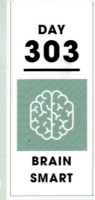

DAY 303

BRAIN SMART

Could the answers to your daily dilemmas be in your dreams?

Today, try a dream journal to log your nighttime problem-solving capabilities. Here's how:

1. Begin with something simple, like how to fit an oversize sofa into your overstuffed living room. Slowly work your way up to more intricate problems, like how to resolve a childhood issue with your sister.

2. Make the question the last thing you think about before nodding off. Sum up your problem in one or two short sentences. If possible, put an object representing the quandary on your bedside table. If not, call to mind a clear image of the issue—just make sure it's the last thing you mull over.

3. Keep a pad of paper and a pen by your bed. Upon waking, take a moment to lie quietly. Glance around the outskirts of your consciousness to see if a dream is lurking. If a fragment comes into your head, gently follow it backward. We usually remember our dreams in reverse. So, like a loose piece of yarn, a dream may unravel if you tug gently on one end.

Dream research has even revealed how long it takes the brain to sort out those answers—a solution to a problem can take a week or longer to surface.

What's a problem you can dream on tonight?

_____

_____

DAY 304

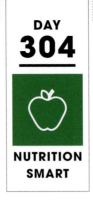

NUTRITION SMART

Plan now to prep a meal this coming Sunday (or your next day off). Make the commitment for the next week, and odds are you'll feel good about cooking healthy, homemade food for yourself—and saving yourself some mental energy on busy weeknights. Ideas:

- **Whole-wheat pasta** with veggies
- **Oatmeal** breakfast bars
- **Hard-boiled eggs**
- **Roasted whole chicken**
- **Raw crunchy veggies:** carrots, celery, radish and bell peppers
- **Roasted veggies:** onion, mushroom, bell pepper, sweet potato

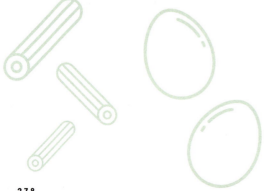

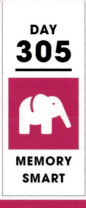

DAY 305

MEMORY SMART

Today, get super-specific when trying to remember a task. To remember to stop at the grocery store on your way home from work or before picking up the kids at soccer practice, make your intention as specific as possible. Don't just tell yourself that you're going to stop at the store. Instead, say that you plan to turn right on Main Street and then turn left into the store parking lot at the second stop sign.

Even when you're not thinking of them, these types of prospective memories (remembering to do something in the future) often stay in your subconscious mind and then pop up when they're needed, research reveals. The system doesn't always work perfectly, though, especially if you have a lot of things on your mind. Making sure the right piece of info pops into your brain at the right time is a phenomenal requirement on the system. So the more detail you can add to the memory, the better, since it gives your mind more ways to trigger the recall of that memory.

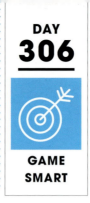

DAY
306

GAME SMART

Rebus Puzzles

What message is each of these word pictures trying to send?

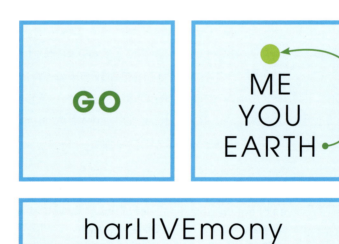

GO

ME
YOU
EARTH

harLIVEmony

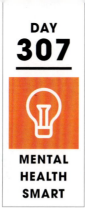

DAY 307

MENTAL HEALTH SMART

Brief mindfulness meditation sessions can improve memory and attention, ease anxiety, and even deepen personal relationships, research suggests. Try this technique, called the Body Scan. Set aside 10 to 20 minutes, and lie comfortably on your back, side, or stomach with your eyes closed.

Beginning with the toes of your left foot, focus on any sensations (tingling, warmth) that you feel there. Now imagine your breath traveling down to your toes, then back up and out through your nose. Slowly move up your left leg, focusing on sensations you encounter and directing your focus to your ankle, shin, knee, and thigh.

Repeat the sequence with your right leg, and then move through your lower back, abdomen, upper back, chest, shoulders, and both arms. Next, move to your neck, throat, face, the back of your head, and finally the top of your head. You should also take notice when you don't feel any sensations at all.

How did you feel before the body scan?

___

How do you feel afterward?

___

DAY 308 — BODY SMART

Today, don't just try to remind yourself to stand during phone calls—force yourself. Place your phone on a high shelf at your desk. Take calls on your cellphone whenever you can, and pace while you talk. And for those drawn-out Zoom meetings, take advantage of all that extra time. Turn off your camera and try to sneak in a few squats or reps with free weights while you listen.

DAY 309 — GAME SMART

How Many? Count the number of squares you can find in this image.

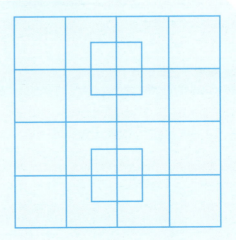

DAY 310 **BRAIN SMART**

Tonight, boost brainpower with a blockbuster. Grab a friend and hit a movie theater, and then go out for dinner afterward to talk about the flick. The deep or innovative thinking that often arises from discussing a good film helps strengthen your mind because it involves reasoning and attention skills. After the credits roll, discuss the movie's themes as if they were in a book you've read. (Don't just rehash the plot.)

DAY 311 **NUTRITION SMART**

Eat an extra clove or two of garlic. It may be bad for your breath, but garlic is packed with vitamin B6, manganese, and other natural elements proven to reduce inflammation and platelet buildup in your blood and arteries, research finds. That's good news for your heart and mind: The increased blood flow to your brain may also ward off age-related cognitive decline. Garlic breath? Brush and floss.

DAY 312 — MEMORY SMART

Name It

Write down as many varieties of fruit as you can remember in 1 minute. How did you do?

_____

_____

_____

_____

_____

_____

_____

_____

_____

_____

DAY 313 — GAME SMART

A plane crashes on the border of the U.S. and Canada. Where do they bury the survivors?

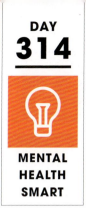

DAY 314 — MENTAL HEALTH SMART

Today, try to summon a sense of purpose. Knowing what gives your life meaning and what gives you a sense of purpose is the path to finding your happiness. In one study, researchers discovered that people with high "purpose in life" scores also enjoyed a strong sense of happiness and satisfaction.

How do you find or rediscover yours? Over time, your purpose can change or even get lost. Try this: Think back to a period of your life when you felt satisfied and fulfilled. What were you doing? Who were you with? Ask yourself what and who matters to you most, and write your thoughts below.

The answers will program your personal GPS. The next step you take—with intent and purpose—will be on the true path to lasting happiness.

_____
_____
_____
_____

| DAY **315** | | **BODY SMART** |

Make a note to ask your doctor about your thyroid or vitamin deficiencies at your next physical. Brain fog could signal a vitamin or hormone deficiency, especially if you've also been feeling unusually tired. One possible culprit is hypothyroidism, a condition caused by low thyroid hormone levels. If you have this deficiency, your metabolism slows down, resulting in reduced blood flow and cellular function in various parts of your brain.

| DAY **316** | | **GAME SMART** |

Calendar Riddle
If the day before yesterday is the 19th, what is the day after tomorrow?

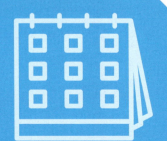

DAY 317

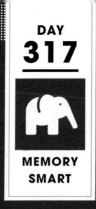

MEMORY SMART

If you've been struggling with reading the news online lately, try (re)turning to print. A meta-analysis of 54 studies found that people who read print pages instead of screen text had better retention of information, which was especially true when time constraints and information-heavy texts were involved. **Not so much time to read today? Pick up an old-fashioned print newspaper.**

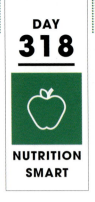

DAY 318 — NUTRITION SMART

Try this fruit- and nut-spiked treat in the morning, or whenever you need the vitamins and omega-3s your inner brainiac craves.

Berry Flax Oats

Boil 1 cup water.

Add ¼ cup steel-cut oats. Cook, stirring, for 25 minutes, until the oatmeal is soft

Reduce the heat to low and cook for 3 more minutes, stirring constantly.

Add ¼ cup fat-free milk, a tablespoon of slivered almonds, ⅓ cup fresh or frozen blueberries, and a teaspoon of ground flaxseed.

Mix and serve.

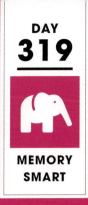

DAY 319

MEMORY SMART

Try applying one of the reading techniques you've learned in this book to an online article. (We don't mean a print article as on Day 317.) How do they compare? Do you remember more one way than another, or do you find no difference at all? Write down your impressions below.

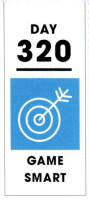

DAY 320 — GAME SMART

Word Ladder

How many steps will it take to get to DONE? Change just one letter at a time—we've done the first one for you.

PLAN   _____

PLAY   _____

_____   _____

_____   _____

_____   DONE

DAY 321

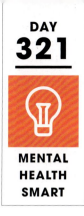

MENTAL HEALTH SMART

Create a transition space in your home. After a day at work or doing errands, pause for a transition as you enter the house. Keep a pair of comfy slippers in the entryway so you can shed your business shoes and persona. Or light a scented candle in the living room and take a minute to enjoy the fragrance. Brainstorm the space where you'll transition between the outside world and your inside world, and describe a routine below:

___

Bonus move: Place an empty jar by the door for your pocket change. When the jar gets full, give the money to a favorite charity. You'll declutter your pockets and purse while also keeping in touch with the things you value.

DAY 322 BRAIN SMART

It's time to teach yourself something new again! Use online videos to learn a new dance step or yoga pose. Learning new ways to move your body should also require your brain to work in new ways.

DAY 323 GAME SMART

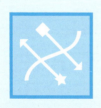

Mirror, Mirror
Can you determine which image in the bottom row is a reflection, as if in a pond or a mirror, of the one on top?

A

B

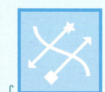
C

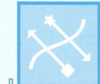
D

DAY 324 **BRAIN SMART**

Today, show your work. Relying on your phone's calculator to determine tips at restaurants robs you of a chance to build and maintain brain pathways. Mathematical skills need to be reinforced, or your brain will eliminate neural connections that aren't in use. Try doing mental math the next time you're out to eat. Or if you have to, jot down your calculations on a napkin.

DAY 325 **NUTRITION SMART**

Try borscht (traditional Eastern European beet soup) or add beets to a salad. You can't beat beets, it turns out. Beets are rich in nitrate, which is converted to nitric oxide in the blood. Nitric oxide relaxes blood vessels throughout the body, enhancing blood flow. The more blood that reaches your brain, the sharper you'll be.

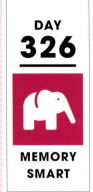

DAY 326

MEMORY SMART

Today, try navigating

to a destination you regularly visit, but without using GPS or other direction-finding software. Relying on GPS can be a missed opportunity—you're wasting the chance to build areas of your brain that control spatial skills. In one study of London cabbies who navigated the city's tangled streets without technological assistance, the cabbies' brains grew as they learned their way around.

Another study

found that people in a driving simulation built more accurate maps of the route in their minds than did people who simply followed navigation guidance.

DAY 327 GAME SMART

Riddle
What's lighter than a feather, but can't be held for long by even the strongest person?

DAY 328 MENTAL HEALTH SMART

Worried? Plan a 30-minute session to deal with all your worries. Then, when anxious thoughts come up, try jotting them down to deal with them at the appointed "worry hour." Most people think they won't be able to postpone that long, but find that this strategy works. A thought might feel urgent at noon, but then 4 p.m. comes and you're not as concerned. You'll think more clearly without worries in the way.

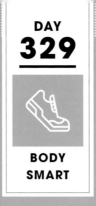

DAY 329

BODY SMART

FLOSS

at least once today. If the sound of a dentist's drill doesn't motivate you to brush and floss regularly, maybe this info will: An emerging body of evidence links dental health to brain health and suggests that gum problems may raise your risk of dementia. So be proactive: Brush twice a day for 2 minutes, and floss at least once a day.

  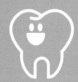

Visit your dentist at least once a year for a cleaning and checkup. If your gums bleed regularly when you brush or floss, see your dentist now.

DAY 330

GAME SMART

Untangle the picture
Choose the four images that, together, create the one on top.

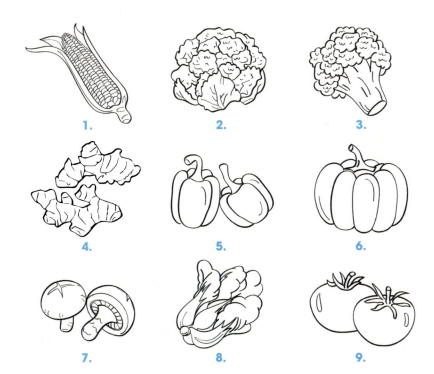

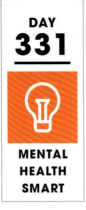

DAY 331

MENTAL HEALTH SMART

Your brain is a laughing matter.

Humor yields important neuropsychological benefits—it improves your mood, exercises your brain, masks pain, and even strengthens your bonds with the people who share a good chuckle with you. A good knee-slapper also produces a chemical reaction that instantly elevates your mood, reduces pain and stress, and boosts immunity. (And as you know, both stress and pain can suppress immunity).

A few ways to add a smile or two:

- **Keep an eye out for** the unexpectedly silly side of daily life to combat negative thoughts.

- **Keep your evening entertainment light** by reading a comic novel or watching a funny show.

- **Reframe unpleasant situations** with humor.

DAY 332

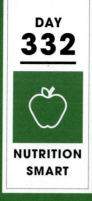

NUTRITION SMART

HAVE AT LEAST 1 TABLESPOON OF OLIVE OIL WITH YOUR MEAL TODAY,

whether in a smoothie, salad dressing, or pasta. In an animal study, researchers discovered that consuming extra virgin olive oil may safeguard memory and learning ability, as well as reduce the formation of 2 Alzheimer's markers (amyloid-beta plaques and neurofibrillary tangles). Though the exact mechanism is unclear, the antioxidant oleocanthal found in the oil may play a role.

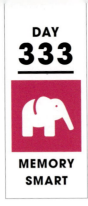

DAY 333

MEMORY SMART

Today, pay close attention

to one item of clothing someone is wearing. Note the colors, patterns, texture, and more, and jot down 4 details below. Later this evening, try to recall them all and check your notes to see how well you did.

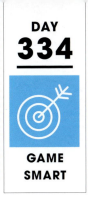

DAY 334

GAME SMART

Jumble Unscramble the words below and then use the letters in blue to discover what we're all about.

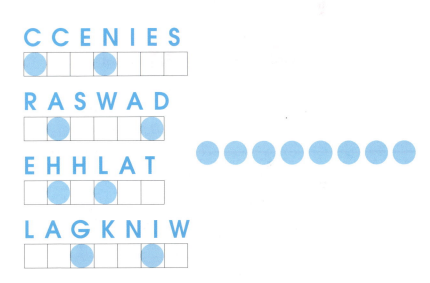

C C E N I E S

R A S W A D

E H H L A T

L A G K N I W

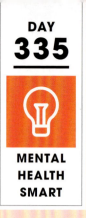

DAY 335

MENTAL HEALTH SMART

Some of the world's most beautiful places are accessible only on foot, and following a trail to get somewhere can be absorbing, inspiring, and humbling. Head out to a trail and start walking, whether it's for a quick 30-minute stroll or a solid half-day hike. You can find a footpath in a nearby local, state, or national park through the American Hiking Society. Its website (americanhiking.org) has a handy "Hikes Near You" tool.

DAY 336

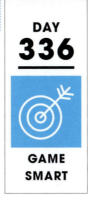

GAME SMART

Rebus Puzzles

Can you figure out what each of these word pictures is trying to say?

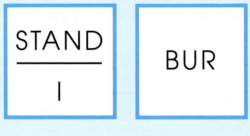

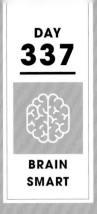

DAY 337

BRAIN SMART

Write a "stop doing" list:

It's hard to fire up your brain with new things when you're just trying to get through the same daily rush-rush routine. What could you eliminate from your life now that would allow more room for a new brain-building activity? You could "stop doing" doomscrolling through bad news, and instead make time to read a book. Instead of spending hours jealously reading Facebook posts, you could practice photography skills. Make the 2 lists below.

Stop Doing

_____

_____

_____

_____

Start Doing

_____

_____

_____

_____

DAY 338

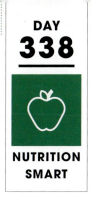

NUTRITION SMART

Eat a plum.

These stone fruits are a good source of anthocyanins, which are powerful antioxidants that give them their purple-red color and play a role in brain function and motor control. Research has even found a possible link between plums and improved cognition. Enjoy 1 to 2 servings a day of deeply hued produce, such as plums, berries, pomegranates, red cabbage, or red grapes.

> **SWEET AND SAVORY GREENS:** Toss 6 plums (quartered) and 4 heads baby bok choy (halved) with 1 Tbsp olive oil. Grill until lightly charred and tender, 1 to 3 min. per side. Toss with 2 tsp each of low-sodium soy sauce, rice vinegar, grated fresh ginger, and 2 scallions (thinly sliced).

| DAY **339** | | **MEMORY SMART** |

If you lose your keys often, say out loud the spot where you're dropping them. That creates a more distinctive memory to call on later. An alternative: Use a key-tracking device called a Tile.

| DAY **340** | | **GAME SMART** |

Find the Finish
What 5-letter word can be added to each of the words below to create all new words?

COUNTER   PIN
NEEDLE   VIEW

DAY 341

MENTAL HEALTH SMART

Enhance your mindfulness today.

Do you ever feel like the noise in your head interferes with your focus and concentration? Learning to be mindful of the details in the world around you can strengthen your ability to sustain attention. (It's an effective stress buster too.)

Take a 5-minute stroll in a familiar place. But instead of letting your thoughts drift to worries and daily concerns, focus on what's going on around you. At the end of your walk, write down 5 things you saw that you'd never noticed before. List them here.

_____

_____

_____

_____

_____

_____

DAY 342 **BODY SMART**

Working on your balance throughout life will mean that by your later years, when your balance gets rockier, you'll just need to maintain what you already have instead of starting from scratch. Try these do-anywhere balance boosters:

1. Stand on one foot while brushing your teeth or waiting in line at the grocery store.

2. Walk heel to toe for 20 steps when grabbing the mail or heading to your car.

3. Stand on your tiptoes while washing dishes or blow-drying your hair.

DAY 343 **BRAIN SMART**

Find a website that offers a daily puzzle. For example, the *New York Times* offers a free daily mini edition of its crossword puzzles online.

DAY 344

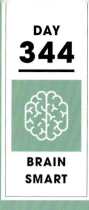

BRAIN SMART

Apply the new knowledge you pick up. When you read an interesting article online, spend 15 minutes thinking about it and how you might apply it to your life. If you and your partner watch a new Netflix series, talk about its message and how it connects with your life, rather than just binge-watching mindlessly. Research shows when people engage in deeper levels of thinking, they increase by 30% the speed of connectivity across the brain's central executive network, which is where decision-making, planning, goal-setting, and clear thinking happen.

Write down some of your thoughts here.

_____
_____
_____
_____
_____

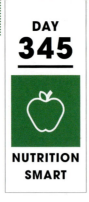

DAY 345

NUTRITION SMART

Sneak this whole-grain goodness

into your day, in the morning or for lunch.

Cream of Bulgur Wheat with Apples
Mix **1 cup cooked bulgur wheat** with **1 cup fat-free milk** and **¼ cup chopped red apple** and heat for 2 min. in the microwave, stirring halfway through. Top with a **pinch of cinnamon, 1 tsp honey, 2 Tbsp** plus **1 tsp slivered almonds,** and ¼ cup chopped red apple.

DAY 346

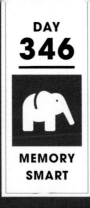

MEMORY SMART

You've accomplished so much in the past year. Now, test your memory with a friend's help.

1. Ask a friend to write down 13 words. (Nouns that are unrelated to one another are best.)

2. Have the person read the list to you, slowly enough for it to take about 25 seconds.

3. Immediately recall as many words as you can and tell them to your friend. Repeat the same process, with the same words, twice more.

4. Take a break and let yourself get distracted (e.g., check email, run a quick errand).

5. After 20 minutes, meet up with your friend and see how many of the 13 words you remember.

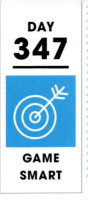

DAY 347

GAME SMART

DIY Math

Put in the proper symbols (+, -, x, ÷) so the solution to each problem is correct. (Do each calculation in order from left to right.)

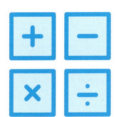

A 3 _ 4 _ 5 = **7**

B 3 _ 4 _ 5 _ 6 = **12**

C 3 _ 4 _ 5 _ 6 _ 7 = **17**

DAY 348

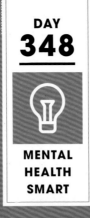

MENTAL HEALTH SMART

The next time you see dirty dishes in the sink,

do them by hand instead of loading the dishwasher. You could lower your stress by up to 27% and feel up to 25% more inspired, one study suggests. The trick is to wash them mindfully: View the task as an experience, not a chore. Focus on little things—the temperature of the water, the smell of the soap, the smooth feel of the dishes.

Increase the zen by using a citrus- or lavender-scented soap: Both smells have been shown to calm the mind. And don't stress if it takes a while to master. Being mindful doesn't mean you have to have a completely clear mind. Even if your mind wanders a thousand times, bring your attention back to the present moment each time.

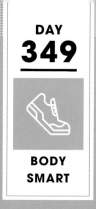

DAY 349

BODY SMART

Make a note to ask your health care provider

to check your hormone levels. A series of hazy days in the mental forecast could be a sign that menopause is near. Midlife brain fog is very real: One study found that women between ages 40 and 60 have trouble staying focused on tricky tasks, and may stumble with something called working memory, which helps you do things like adding up numbers in your head. Hormones shape the brain, so it would make sense for vacillating estrogen levels to cause shifts in cognition, too.

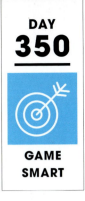

DAY 350 — GAME SMART

Letter Tree

Which letter belongs at the top?

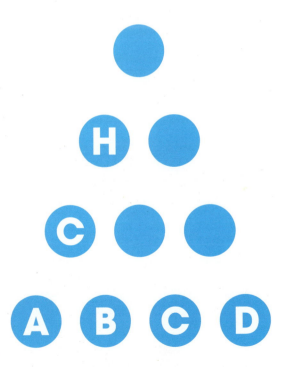

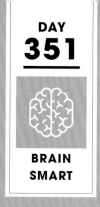

DAY 351

BRAIN SMART

Try something new. Anything new.

If you're not challenging your brain with new places and information, your memory suffers, U.K. research reveals. Familiar activities allow your noodle to lapse into autopilot. But novelty—whether you're exploring a new hiking trail, trying a new food, or solving a tough Sudoku puzzle—can stimulate your brain and memory, the study (and plenty of others) shows.

What one new thing will you do today?

DAY 352

NUTRITION SMART

Like cells throughout your body, brain cells can suffer damage from rogue molecules known as free radicals. Antioxidants come to your defense by disarming those free radicals. These 10 foods have the greatest concentration of antioxidants by weight (in descending order). See how many different categories you can consume today:

- ☐ Blackberries
- ☐ Walnuts
- ☐ Strawberries
- ☐ Artichokes
- ☐ Cranberries
- ☐ Coffee
- ☐ Raspberries
- ☐ Pecans
- ☐ Blueberries
- ☐ Ground cloves

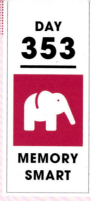

DAY 353

MEMORY SMART

SNIFF

some rosemary: This spice rack staple can be used to improve your memory. The smell of rosemary essential oil may improve the prospective memory of people over age 65, some research suggests.

Prospective memory is the ability to remember specific events and tasks that will happen in the future—like your 2 .p.m. appointment or your partner's birthday. (By contrast, retrospective memory is your recall of the past.)

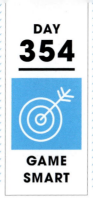

DAY
354

GAME SMART

Same or Different?

In this set of images, find three pairs, one trio, and one that doesn't match any of the others.

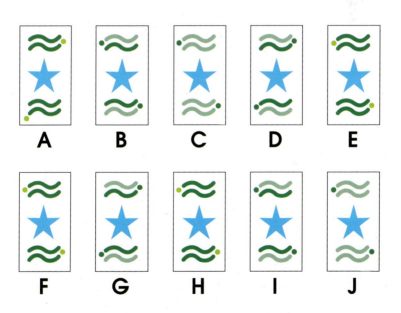

DAY 355 **MENTAL HEALTH SMART**

Lower the thermostat and turn your bedroom into a chilly, dark space for a better night's sleep. The ideal temperature for snoozing is about 61°F, according to a study in the journal *Sleep*. At that temperature, people slept up to 30 minutes longer and reported being more alert the next day than when they slept in a room that was about 10 degrees warmer.

DAY 356 **BRAIN SMART**

Switch to round-bottom tennis shoes (also called "rocker bottom" shoes) once a week, or swap out tennies for sandals when walking for exercise today. Moving in shoes you're not used to wearing forces you to pay more attention to your coordination and gets those brain synapses firing.

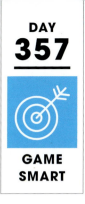

Missing Piece

Which puzzle piece will fit?

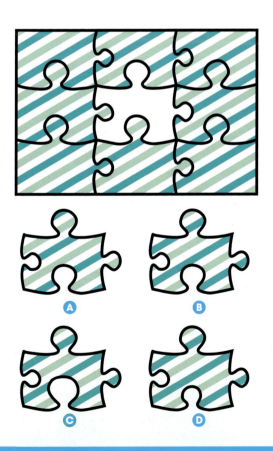

DAY 358

BRAIN SMART

Today, grab a pencil and sketch out your to-do list.

Illustrating something you don't want to forget may be even more beneficial than writing it down, research suggests. You're more likely to recall your sketch later, because drawing employs motor, word, and visual skills. Plus, fully engaging in an activity such as drawing eases stress—and stress hinders brainpower. Try it below with something you need to remember: your grocery list, your daily tasks, or calls you need to make.

DAY 359

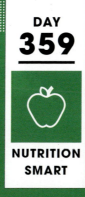

NUTRITION SMART

Fuel with folate.

Without folate, you risk depression, short-term memory loss, and dementia, a Canadian study indicates. While folate deficiency isn't common, you can find folate in these foods:

- Spinach
- Asparagus
- Peanuts
- Broccoli
- Avocados
- Oranges
- Kidney beans
- Brussels sprouts
- Enriched breakfast cereals and flour products

| DAY **360** | | MEMORY SMART |

Here's a chance to practice what you've learned in the past year. Read this, and then close the book and see how much you remember.

Andrea Ingram takes the 7:30 a.m. train to work every weekday from Bloomfield Station, near her home in New Jersey. One morning, as the train passed through a deserted area just outside the town of Glen View, Andrea noticed a dog wandering near the tracks. She quickly alerted the conductor, Mr. Greenwood, who contacted the local authorities. The next morning, Andrea brought her three sons to the animal shelter where the dog had been taken. The dog, a poodle mix, was healthy and appeared to enjoy playing with the boys. Andrea's middle son, Henry, returned 2 days later and brought the dog a toy bone. After 1 month, the authorities had not found the dog's owners, so Andrea and her children adopted the dog. They named her Tracks.

| DAY **361** | | GAME SMART |

Word Scramble

Can you make at least 5 five-letter words from the word **PREVENTION**?

324

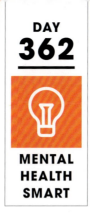

DAY 362

MENTAL HEALTH SMART

Research shows that social support is the single greatest predictor of happiness, health, and longevity, all of which are related to resilience. The right people can act as a buffer for stress, countering hormones such as cortisol that can hamper your ability to cope. Here's how to think about who's in your life:

AVOID THOSE WHO leave you feeling emotionally exhausted after you talk to them.

FIND FOLKS WHO give as much as you do or allow you to chill: You'll have more energy to face your own challenges when support goes both ways.

AVOID THOSE WHO are reluctant to try new things.

FIND FOLKS WHO inspire you: Doing novel activities forges new brain connections, which come in handy when you have a setback and need to adapt fast.

AVOID THOSE WHO constantly complain and pick things apart.

FIND FOLKS WHO are not cynical or negative. Cynicism places limits on you and others, and when building resilience, it's more useful to focus on the possibility of growth.

AVOID THOSE WHO see you frozen in time.

FIND FOLKS WHO help you visualize your way forward: Seek out friends who give you the confidence to break old patterns.

DAY 363

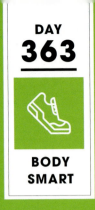

BODY SMART

Changing the direction you walk—forward, backward, or sideways—keeps your mind alert, revs up your calorie burn, and activates some often-underused muscles, such as your outer and inner thighs. This routine is best done on a school track. (Most are ¼ mile around.) **Check out the workout below.**

Lap 1: Start at the beginning of the curved part of the track. To warm up, walk as you normally would for a full lap.

Lap 2: Turn sideways so your right foot is in front. Sidestep or shuffle around the curved part of the track. Walk backward on the straight section. Sidestep through the next curve with your left foot in front. Walk forward on the straight section.

Lap 3: Repeat Lap 2, walking sideways, backward, sideways, and forward.

Lap 4: Walk forward, slowing your pace to cool down.

This is a 1-mile walk if you use a ¼-mile track. You can do more laps to extend it, or work up to doing half or even full laps of each type of walking.

DAY 364

GAME SMART

Logic Puzzle

Jack, Jessie, Mack, Mary, and Xavier were in a 5-person race. Jack came in ahead of 2 runners but behind the other 2. Xavier came in right after Mack, and Jessie came in right after Mary. Xavier came in after Mary.

Who won the race?

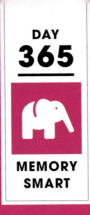

DAY 365

MEMORY SMART

Write down 10 things you've taken away in the past year that you've tried once—and liked so much you've made a habit.

ANSWERS

Day 5: Connect the Dots

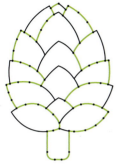

Day 15: Cryptogram
Prevention is the best medicine.

Day 19: Mystery Cube
A

Day 26: Symbols Brain Booster
From left:
1st symbol: 12
2nd symbol: 16
3rd symbol: 11

Day 29: Fill in the Blanks
Row 1: 26, 31, 36
Row 2: 34, 40, 46
Row 3: L, N, P
Row 4: 8, H
Row 5: **, +

Day 33: Berry Good at Math
Strawberry: 5
Blueberry: 7
Blackberry: 9

Day 36: Brainteaser
S, O, N (September, October, and November) are the next in sequence. The sequence is the first letter of the months of the year.

Day 40: Math Square
Square: top left = 8,
Top right = 1, Bottom left = 3, Bottom right = 5

Day 43: Middlemen
board, light, time, apple, out

Day 47: Crack the Code
D; masterful

Day 50: Rebus Rally
BIG BAD WOLF
SLOW DOWN
READ BETWEEN THE LINES
CLEVER AFTERTHOUGHT
WARM UP
EGGS OVER EASY
KEEP IN TOUCH
GOOD AFTERNOON
CORNER TABLE
LESSER OF TWO EVILS

Day 54: Word Sequence
A: Everybody (the first letter is E, following words that begin with A, B, C, and D; the word is 9 letters long, following words that are 1, 3, 5, and 7 letters long)

Day 55: Cipher
Great job. Your brain is trained.

Day 61: Maze

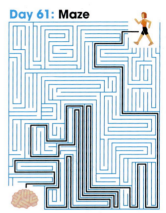

Day 68: Cryptogram
You must do the thing you think you cannot do.

Day 71: Missing Pieces
A

Day 75: Phrase Anagram
They see. Twelve plus one. Can't rely on it.

Day 81: Riddle
A keyboard

Day 100: Puzzle
D

Day 106: Resale Riddle
Yes, $20 (to solve, start at $0, so when she buys the lamp, she is out $40).

Day 113: Number Wheel
6, 4

Day 117: Family Riddle
You are Anna's daughter.

Day 120: Group Game
7 groups

Day 124: DIY Cube
A

Day 131: Message
Get in great shape by using this book. Surprise yourself and your friends with your powers of deductive reasoning. Seem familiar? Perhaps you or your kids like to text message.

Day 134: Rebus Puzzles
No U-turn, play on words, top secret

Day 138: Cryptogram
The greatest wealth is health.

Day 141: Connect The Dots

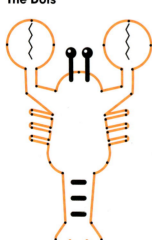

Day 145: Find the Difference
348 (for the others, the first two digits can be multiplied to create the final digit or digits)

Day 152: Number Pattern
19 (these are prime numbers between 10 and 30)

Day 155: Trivia
Mount Everest

Day 159: Number Riddle
41 years ago

Day 162: Triangles
13

Day 166: Mystery Word Search
The words are banana, broccoli, kale, quinoa, salmon, walnut

Day 169: Math Logic
80

Day 173: Visual Math
Apple = 30
strawberry = 10
orange = 20

Day 183: Fill in The Blanks
Row 1 = 23, 27, 31
Row 2 = 37, 44, 51
Row 3 = P, S, V
Row 4 = 7, G
Row 5 = ff, i

Day 187: Word Finder
Remaining letters spell HEALTHIER.

Day 190: Cryptogram
Grow old along with me! The best is yet to be. (Robert Browning) Each letter in the quote is replaced by the second letter that comes after it in the alphabet.

Day 194: Coded Message
Act as if what you do makes a difference. It does.

Day 201: Shape Sudoku

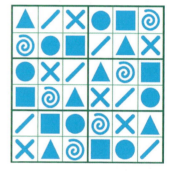

Day 204: Do the Math
177-77

Day 208: Missing Letters
ART

Day 210: Sequencing Skills
20

Day 218: Reading + Math
4 (25–26 and 41–42 are each on the same sheet of paper).

Day 222: Missing Piece
A

Day 229:
Mystery Word Search
Farro, rice, quinoa; kale, spinach, arugula; plum, pear, kiwi

Day 239: Rebus Rally
1. Eggs over easy
2. Buy low, sell high
3. Scotch on the rocks

Day 253: Add to the Top
88

Day 257: Odd One Out
7

Day 260: Missing Math
A: +, ÷, x. B: -, x, +. C: -, x, x. D: x, +, -.

Day 264: Missing Piece
A

Day 267:
Spot the Symbol
(from left) 14, 25, 14

Day 274: What's Missing
B

Day 278:
Missing Number Square
47 (pair the first digit from the number on the left with the second digit from the number on the right)

Day 281: Building Blocks
B

Day 285: Cryptogram
"To be, or not to be: That is the question." Each numeral is the number of the letter in the alphabet, plus one.

Day 288: Multiply This
483 x 12 = 5,796

Day 295: Bird's Eye View
C

Day 299: Line Drawing
Hint: Start at the top left corner of the square and go left/down, then right/down, then at the bottom left corner of the square, go up, then diagonal right/down.

Day 302:
Order by Number
942

Day 306: Rebus Puzzles
Go green. Put the earth first. Live in harmony.

Day 309: How Many?
40 (Don't forget the 3 x 3 square!)

Day 313: Riddle
You don't bury the SURVIVORS!

Day 316:
Calendar Riddle
The 23rd.

Day 320: Word Ladder
We did it in 10 steps.

Day 323: Mirror, Mirror
C

Day 327: Riddle
Your breath.

Day 330: Untangle the Picture
3, 4, 6, 9

Day 334: Jumble
Science, awards, health, walking. Final answer: Wellness.

Day 336: Rebus Puzzles
I understand, back up, scrambled eggs

Day 340: Find the Finish
Point

Day 347: DIY Math
A: x, -. B: +, -, x. C: x, x, ÷, +.

Day 350: Letter Tree
T (convert each letter to its corresponding number in the alphabet, then add the two adjacent numbers to determine the letter above each pair).

Day 354: Same or Different? Pairs: B and I, C and J, D and G; Trio: E, F, H; Single: A.

Day 357:
Missing Piece
B

Day 361:
Word Scramble
Event, overt, preen, print, toner.

Day 364:
Logic Puzzle
Mary

Sources List
Thanks to these experts, institutions, and journals for their brain health insights.

Experts
Aaron Nelson, Ph.D., Adam Borland, Psy.D., Adam Hanley, Allison Childress, Ph.D., R.D.N., CSSD, Amy Chan, Ph.D., Anil Nigam, M.D., Anita Sanchez, Ph.D., Barry Jordan, Brent Masel, M.D., Brent Roberts, Ph.D., Brian Fligor, Sc.D., Brooke Lea, Ph.D., Carolyn Yoon, Ph.D., Catherine Harrison, Ph.D., Cynthia Green, Ph.D., Daisy Fancourt, Dale E. Bredesen, M.D., Dara Schwartz, Deborah Cracknell, Ph.D., Deirdre Barrett, Ph.D., Don Kuiken, Ph.D., Eileen Luders, Ph.D., Elaine Chin, M.D., Elizabeth Zelinski, Ph.D., Emeran Mayer, M.D., Emily Pronin, Ph.D., Fran Walfish, Psy.D., Frances Kaplan, G. William Domhoff, Ph.D., Gail Saltz, M.D., Gary L. Altman, CRC, HTR, Gary Small, M.D., Gena Glickman, Ph.D., Gregory J. O'Shanick, M.D., Helena Jahncke, Ph.D., Irma Järvelä, M.D., Ph.D., James McGaugh, Ph.D., Jeanne D'Archer, Jennifer McDaniel, Jerlyn Jones, R.D.N., Jessica Flanagan, LSW, John Martin, Ph.D., Jonathan W. Schooler, Ph.D., Jose Biller, M.D., Joy Harden Bradford, Ph.D., Kristin Neff, Ph.D., Laura Murray-Kolb, Ph.D., Laura Vanderkam, Libby Mills, Lisa Mosconi, Ph.D., Lodro Rinzler, Majid Fotuhi, M.D., Marc Berman, Mark Mendell, Ph.D., Martha Clare Morris, Sc.D., Melissa A. St. Hilaire, Ph.D., Michael Breus, Ph.D., Michael Kane, Ph.D., Michele Stanten, Michelle Schoffro Cook, Mike Dow, Psy.D, Ph.D., Mithu Storoni, Paul Nussbaum, Ph.D., Peter Pribis, Phyllis Zee, M.D., Ph.D., Richard Isaacson, M.D., Ritanne Duszak, RD, Robert Emmons, Ph.D., Robert L. Leahy, Robert Lahita, M.D., Ph.D., Robert Madigan, Robert Orford, M.D., Robert S. Wilson, Ph.D., Robin West, Ph.D., Ruth Propper, Ph.D., Sandra Bond Chapman, Ph.D., Sara Mednick, Ph.D., Sarah C. Slayton, Shawna Kaminski, Simon Landry, Ph.D., Sue Fleming, Sung Lee, M.D., Susan Nolen-Hoeksema, Ph.D., Tasneem Bhatia, M.D., Thomas Crook, Ph.D., Timothy S. Church, Ph.D., Tom Shea, Ph.D., Tore Nielsen, Ph.D., Tyler Harrison, W. Chris Winter, M.D., William Howatt, Ph.D.

Universities & Institutions
Albert Einstein College of Medicine, American Chemical Society, American Psychological Association, British Psychological Society's Annual Conference, Center for Genomic Medicine at Kyoto University, Columbia University Irving Medical Center, Deakin University, Florida State University, Harvard University, Johns Hopkins University, King's College London, Lancaster University, Laval University, Loma Linda University, Louisiana State University, Massachusetts General Hospital, Mayo Clinic, National Institute on Aging and Tufts University, North Carolina State University, Northwestern University, Ohio University, Oregon Health & Science University, Oxford University, Rush University, Rush University in Chicago, SUNY and the Lawrence Berkeley National Laboratory, Temple University, U.K.'s National Marine Aquarium, University College London, University of Alabama, University of Exeter, University of Illinois, University of Kentucky, University of Lübeck, University of Michigan, University of North Florida, University of Nottingham, University of Pittsburgh, University of Rochester, University of South Dakota, University of Texas, Dallas, University of Waterloo, University of Wisconsin, University of Wisconsin-Madison, Wellesley College, Wheeling Jesuit University, University of Kentucky College of Medicine

Journals
Alzheimer's & Dementia: The Journal of The Alzheimer's Association, American Journal of Clinical Nutrition, American Journal of Epidemiology, British Psychological Society's Annual Conference, Educational Research Review, Indoor Air, International Journal of Geriatric Psychiatry, JAMA, Journal of Alzheimer's Disease, Journal of Cardiovascular Pharmacology, Journal of Environmental Psychology, Journal of Nutrition, Journal of Sport & Exercise Psychology, Journal of Strength and Conditioning Research, Neurology, New England Journal of Medicine, Nutrients, PLOS ONE, Psychological Science, Sleep, The Journal of Neuroscience

Notes:

Thank You for Purchasing
Get Sharper Every Day

Visit our online store to find more great products from *Prevention* and save 20% off your next purchase.

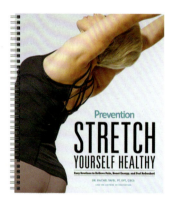

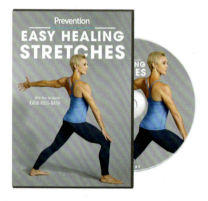

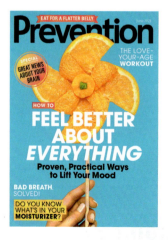

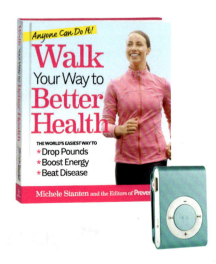

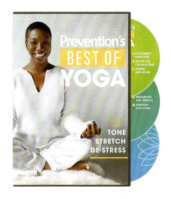
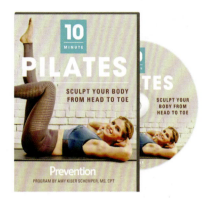
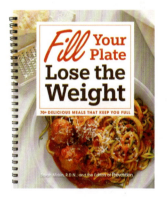
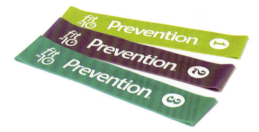

PLEASE ENJOY 20% OFF AT OUR STORE!

20% OFF

USE COUPON CODE **THANKYOU20**

*Exclusions Apply

Shop.Prevention.com